Dysphagia Cookbook For Beginners

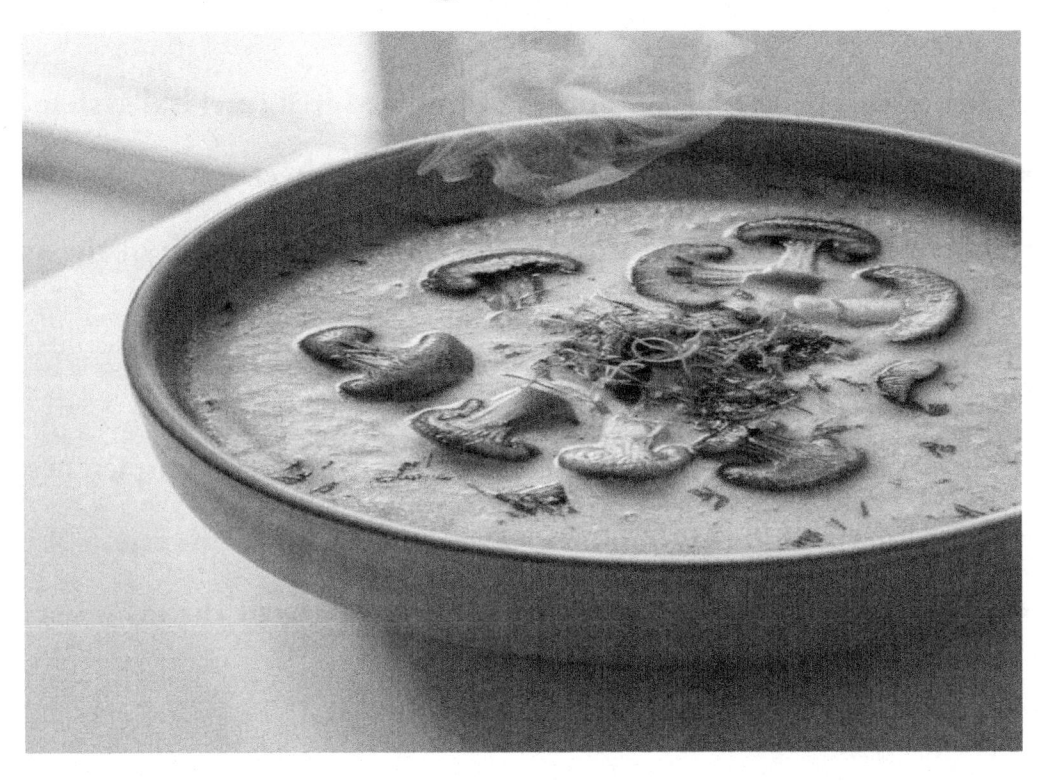

Delicious and Easy to follow recipes for people with chewing and swallowing difficulties

Malon O.Lai

COPYRIGHT © [2024] [**Malon O.Lai***]*
All rights reserved.

No part of this book may be reproduced, stored in a retrieval system, or transmitted in any form or by any means, electronic, mechanical, photocopying, recording, or otherwise, without the prior written permission of the author.

The author has made every effort to ensure the accuracy and completeness of the information contained in this book. However, they assume no responsibility for errors, omissions, or damages resulting from the use of the information contained herein.

Table of Contents

Preface...5

How This Book Can Help...7

Introduction..9

Chapter 1...11

    What is Dysphagia?..11

    Types of Dysphagia..12

    Diagnosis and Treatment Options..16

Chapter 2...19

    Nutritional Needs for Dysphagia Management..............................19

    Overview of Dysphagia Diet Levels (Pureed, Mechanically Altered, Advanced)......21

    Cooking Techniques for Dysphagia..23

    Food Texture Modification...25

    Stocking Your Pantry: Ingredients for Easy Swallowing................27

    Grocery shopping guide...30

Chapter 3...33

    Breakfast Recipes...33

    Smoothies and Thickened Beverages...33

    Soft Pancakes and Modified Eggs..40

    Nutritious Porridges and Cereals..48

Chapter 4: Soups and Stews..57

    Hearty Vegetable Soup...57

    Smooth Cream Soups...66

Chapter 5: Main Dishes 73
    Protein-Rich Purees 73
    Casseroles and One-Pot Meals 92
    Sides and Snacks 101
    Gelatin and Custards 101

Chapter 6: Beverages and Smoothies 111
    Thickened Drinks for Hydration 111
    Flavorful Smoothie and Juice 117

Chapter 7 121
    Meal plan 121

Conclusion 124

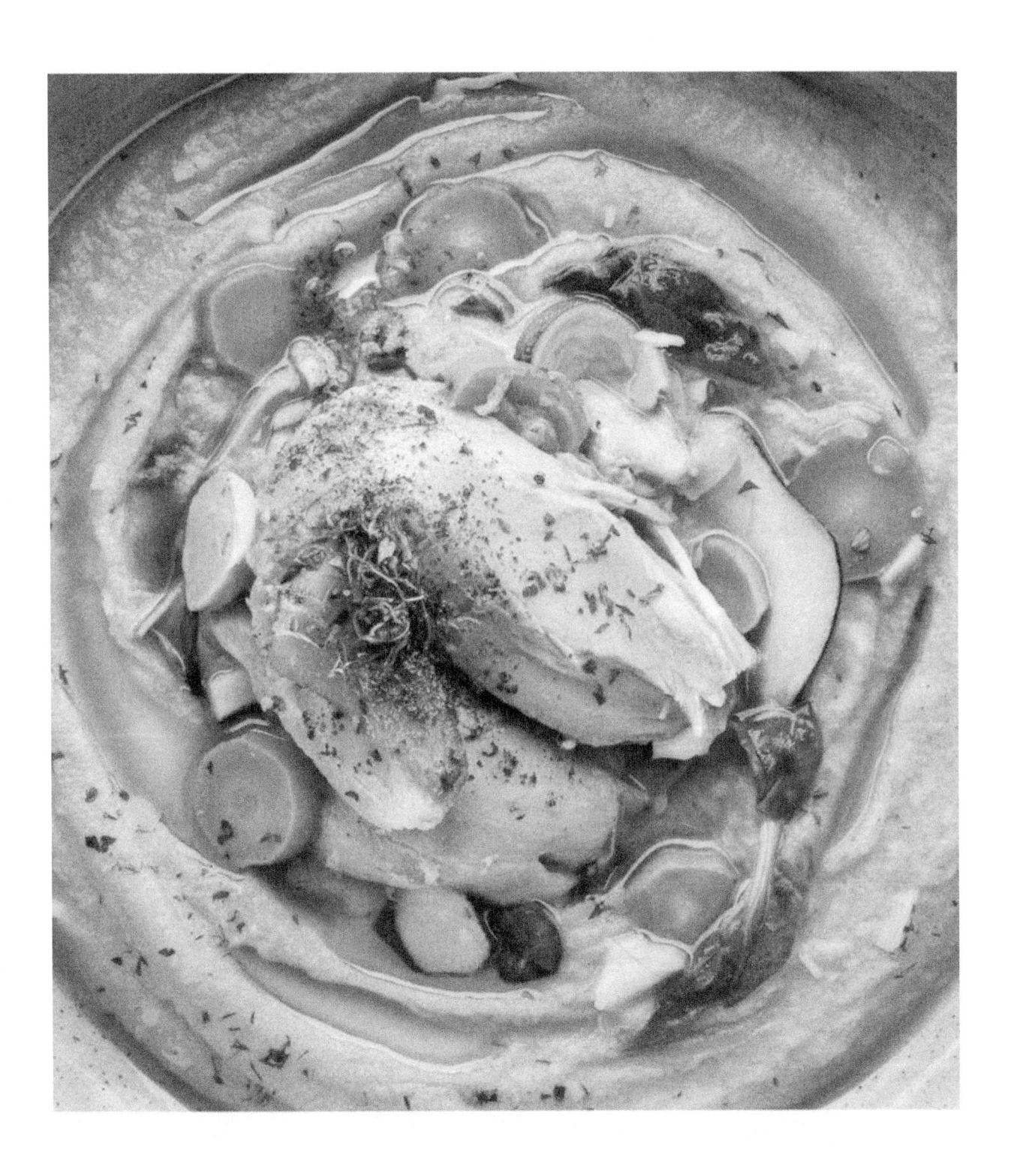

Preface

Welcome and thank you for choosing this cookbook,

As a nutritionist with over a decade of experience working with patients who face daily challenges from various health conditions, dysphagia has emerged as a particularly impactful disorder that affects not just the physical body but also the emotional and social well-being of individuals. The journey into understanding and crafting solutions for dysphagia began several years ago when I encountered my first patient struggling to swallow even the simplest of meals—a warm, soft oatmeal. The fear in her eyes spoke volumes about the challenges she faced at every meal, turning what should be an enjoyable, nourishing experience into a source of anxiety and dread.

Motivated by my patients' struggles and the realization that there were limited resources that addressed the culinary needs of those with dysphagia, I was driven to create this cookbook. My intention was not only to provide recipes that are safe, nutritious, and easy to swallow but also to infuse joy and flavor back into their meals. Food is a fundamental part of our culture and daily pleasure that many of us take for granted. For those dealing with dysphagia, every bite can be a challenge, and I wanted to alleviate that stress as much as possible.

This book is the culmination of years of research, experimentation, and feedback from patients and healthcare professionals. It is designed to be a practical, compassionate guide for individuals newly diagnosed with dysphagia and their caregivers. Through these pages, I aim to offer not just culinary solutions but also a source of comfort and assurance that your dietary needs can be met with creativity and care.

Writing this book has been an emotional journey, both challenging and profoundly rewarding. I've seen firsthand the difference that a thoughtfully prepared meal can make in a patient's demeanor and outlook. It is my sincere hope that this cookbook serves as a valuable tool in managing dysphagia, making mealtime a safer and more enjoyable part of the day. With each recipe, I've aimed to bring a bit of relief, happiness, and normalcy back into the lives of those affected by this challenging condition.

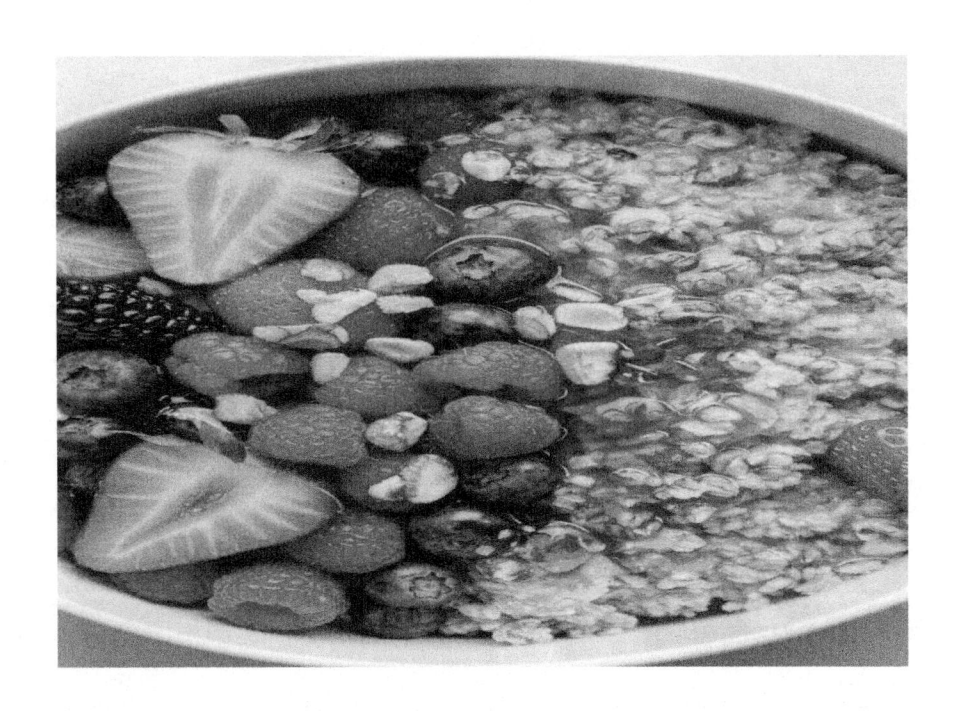

How This Book Can Help

This cookbook is designed to be a practical guide for those newly diagnosed with dysphagia, a condition that can make swallowing difficult and potentially dangerous. Recognizing the challenges that come with this diagnosis, the recipes and tips provided here aim to restore the pleasure of eating while ensuring safety and nutritional balance.

Each recipe in this book has been carefully developed to cater to the specific needs of individuals with swallowing difficulties. The meals are crafted to be easy to swallow, minimizing the risk of choking and aspiration, which are common concerns with dysphagia. To achieve this, textures are modified according to standard dysphagia diet guidelines, ranging from pureed to soft-cooked, ensuring that they meet the required consistency without compromising taste.

Nutrition is a cornerstone of this cookbook. Dysphagia can often lead to reduced food intake, which might result in nutritional deficiencies. This book addresses that risk by offering nutrient-dense recipes that provide essential vitamins, minerals, and proteins, all tailored to be as enjoyable as they are healthful. The recipes also include a variety of ingredients to encourage a balanced diet and incorporate options for all meals of the day, from breakfast smoothies to nourishing dinners.

Also, this cookbook serves as an educational tool, offering insights into the techniques for preparing dysphagia-appropriate meals. It provides guidance on how to thicken liquids, how to modify existing favorite recipes, and how to ensure that food textures are safe yet appetizing. This approach not only aids in maintaining physical health but also supports the emotional and social well-being of those affected by dysphagia. Eating is a social activity, and by enabling safer, more enjoyable meals, this book helps preserve the communal joy of dining with family and friends.

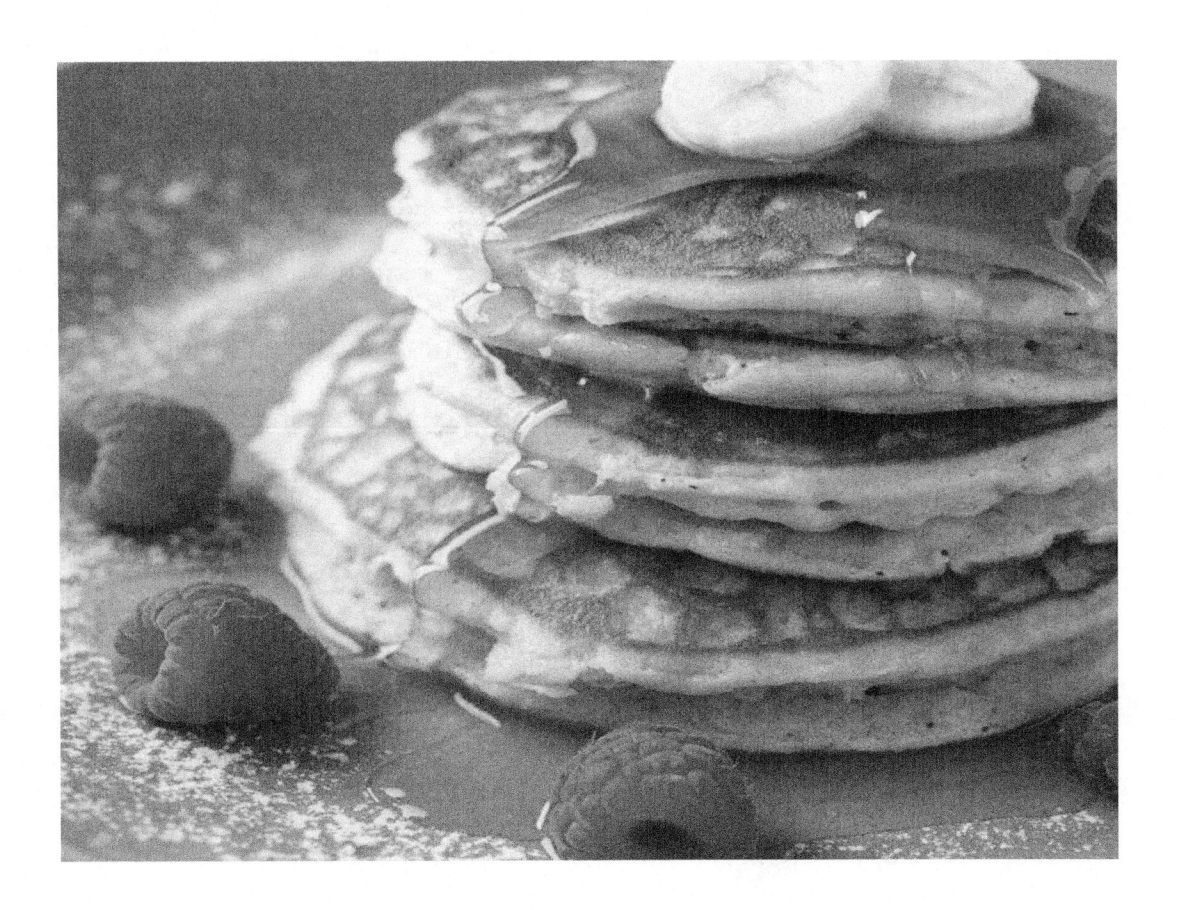

Introduction

Dysphagia, a condition characterized by difficulty in swallowing, can significantly alter daily life and overall health. When someone is diagnosed with dysphagia, simple pleasures like eating a meal can become challenging and sometimes dangerous. This condition may stem from various causes, including neurological disorders, muscular diseases, or structural damage. The impact on daily life is profound as it affects not only the ability to enjoy food but also the social and emotional aspects of dining.

Nutrition plays a pivotal role in managing dysphagia. Ensuring that the body receives adequate nutrients without compromising safety requires careful planning and preparation. Foods must be prepared in a way that minimizes the risk of choking and aspiration, which can lead to pneumonia and other complications. Adapting meals to the appropriate consistency, whether pureed, minced, or soft, helps maintain adequate nutrition and hydration, vital for healing and health.

This cookbook is designed to support you by providing recipes that cater to the nutritional needs and textural requirements unique to dysphagia sufferers. It aims to reintroduce the joy of eating by offering meals that are not only safe and easy to swallow but also flavorful and appealing.

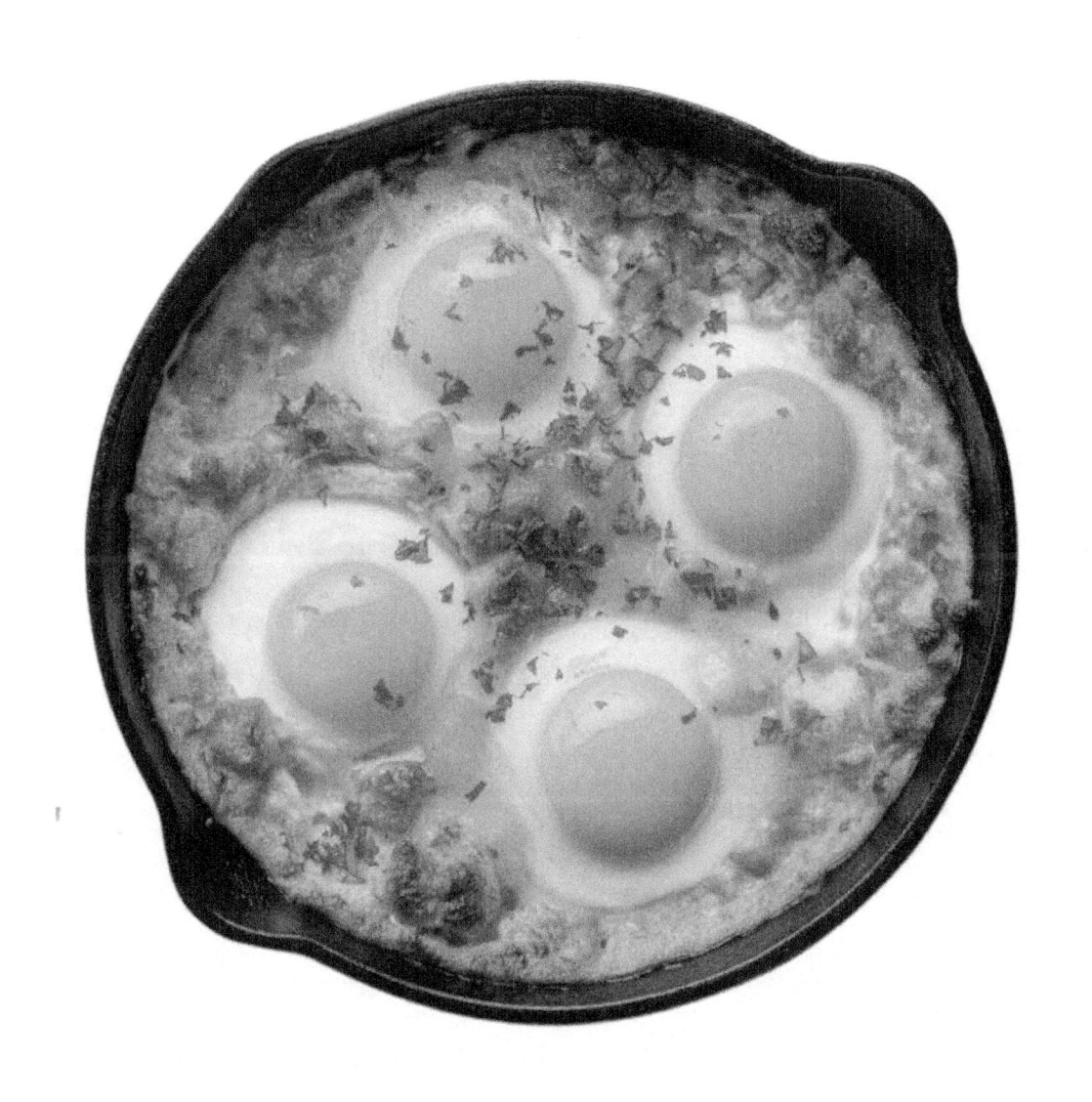

Chapter 1

What is Dysphagia?

Dysphagia is a medical condition that affects the ability to swallow, turning the simple act of eating and drinking into a challenge fraught with anxiety and fear. It can occur at any stage of the swallowing process—from the moment food or liquid is placed in the mouth, through the throat, and down into the esophagus leading to the stomach. For those who suffer from dysphagia, each meal can feel like a daunting obstacle, overshadowed by the threat of choking or aspirating food particles into the lungs, which can lead to serious health complications like pneumonia.

The origins of dysphagia are varied, stemming from neurological disorders like stroke, Parkinson's disease, or multiple sclerosis, from muscular diseases such as muscular dystrophy, or from structural problems caused by cancer or surgery that affect the throat or esophagus. Regardless of the cause, the impact on a person's life is significant and far-reaching. Eating is not only a basic human need but also a pleasure and a social activity that brings people together. Dysphagia can strip away these joys, leading to social isolation and emotional distress, and can complicate the management of nutrition and hydration, essential for overall health and well-being.

For many, the diagnosis of dysphagia begins a journey of adaptation, requiring them to learn new ways to prepare and enjoy food. Liquid consistencies must be thickened, solids pureed or softened, and every bite must be carefully calculated to ensure it can be swallowed safely. This often means long-term changes to diet and lifestyle, which can be overwhelming and disheartening.

However, despite these challenges, a diagnosis of dysphagia also brings with it an opportunity for resilience and innovation in the kitchen. With the right resources, such as a dedicated cookbook tailored to the needs of those with dysphagia, it is possible to reclaim the joy of eating. These resources aim to provide safe, nutritious, and tasty meal options that cater to the altered swallowing abilities, allowing meals to be a source of comfort and enjoyment once again, rather than a source of fear.

Types of Dysphagia

Dysphagia, often perceived as a single condition, actually encompasses various types depending on the location and nature of the swallowing difficulties. At its core, dysphagia can be classified into three main types: oropharyngeal, esophageal, and functional. Each type has distinct causes and manifestations, affecting different parts of the swallowing mechanism.

Oropharyngeal dysphagia refers to problems that occur during the initial phases of swallowing, where the muscles and nerves that help control the mouth and throat are affected. This type of dysphagia is commonly associated with neurological disorders such as stroke, Parkinson's disease, or conditions like multiple sclerosis and ALS, which impair the brain's ability to communicate effectively with the swallowing muscles. People with oropharyngeal dysphagia often have difficulty initiating swallowing, and may cough, choke, or experience nasal regurgitation as food mistakenly enters the nasal passages.

Esophageal dysphagia occurs when the problem lies in the esophagus, the tube that carries food from the mouth to the stomach. This type can be caused by a physical blockage in the esophagus, such as a tumor or a stricture, or by motility disorders. Motility disorders, like achalasia, involve the inability of the esophagus to move food toward the stomach due to abnormal muscle activity. Symptoms often include a sensation of food being stuck in the chest, pain during swallowing, or frequent heartburn and regurgitation of food, especially when lying down.

Functional dysphagia represents a more complex diagnosis where the mechanical process of swallowing is normal but the function is impaired. This type is often diagnosed in individuals who experience sensations of choking and difficulty swallowing without any clear physical or neurological cause. Functional dysphagia can be linked to psychological factors or conditions such as anxiety disorders, where the perception of swallowing difficulty persists even though the swallowing mechanism itself is intact.

Each type of dysphagia requires a specific diagnostic approach and targeted treatment strategies. For oropharyngeal dysphagia, strengthening exercises, changes in food textures, and techniques to enhance swallowing safety are often recommended. Esophageal dysphagia might require procedures to stretch or open the esophagus, or surgery to remove blockages. In cases of functional dysphagia, addressing underlying psychological factors alongside dietary adjustments can be crucial.

Recognizing the type of dysphagia is essential for effective management, ensuring that interventions are appropriately tailored to address the unique challenges faced by each individual, thereby improving their ability to eat safely and comfortably.

Mechanics of Swallowing

Swallowing is a complex process that involves over 50 pairs of muscles and many nerves, functioning in a coordinated effort to move food from the mouth to the stomach. This process is divided into three stages:

1. Oral Phase: This is where the preparation and voluntary control of swallowing begins. Food is chewed and mixed with saliva to form a bolus (a mass of chewed food), and the tongue pushes it to the back of the mouth.

2. Pharyngeal Phase: This involuntary phase begins when the bolus triggers receptors in the back of the throat, initiating a swallowing reflex. The larynx (voice box) closes tightly to prevent aspiration, and the bolus moves into the esophagus.

3. Esophageal Phase: The bolus travels down the esophagus through a series of involuntary muscle contractions known as peristalsis. This phase ends as the bolus enters the stomach through the lower esophageal sphincter.

Causes of Dysphagia

Dysphagia can be caused by problems in any of the above phases, due to various underlying conditions:

- *Neurological Causes*: Damage to the brain or nerves from stroke, Parkinson's disease, or brain injury can disrupt the nerve signals vital for the coordination of the swallowing muscles.
- *Structural Causes*: Cancers of the throat or esophagus, injuries, or congenital anomalies (like a cleft palate) can physically block or narrow the passage used by food.
- *Muscle Disorders*: Conditions like scleroderma or achalasia affect how the muscles of the throat and esophagus function. In scleroderma, tissues harden and lose elasticity, while achalasia involves the failure of the esophagus to open fully at the stomach junction, hindering the passage of food.
- *Infectious and Inflammatory Conditions*: Infections like thrush or conditions like eosinophilic esophagitis that cause inflammation and swelling can also lead to swallowing difficulties.

Complex Symptoms and Their Impacts

The symptoms of dysphagia extend beyond simple difficulty swallowing. They can include:

- *Aspiration*: Perhaps the most dangerous symptom, where food or liquid enters the airways, leading to coughing, choking, and serious lung infections.
- *Dehydration and Malnutrition*: These occur as individuals eat less to avoid the pain and discomfort of swallowing.
- *Psychosocial Impacts*: The challenges of dysphagia can lead to anxiety around meals, social isolation, and a decreased quality of life due to the fear of eating in public or the prolonged duration of meals.

Diagnosis and Treatment Options

Medical tests, therapy, and lifestyle changes

Diagnosing dysphagia typically involves a series of medical tests that help pinpoint the type and cause of the swallowing difficulties. One common diagnostic tool is the barium swallow study, where individuals drink a barium solution that coats the digestive tract, making the swallowing process visible on X-ray images. This test helps in identifying blockages or abnormalities in the esophagus and pharynx. Another essential diagnostic tool is endoscopy, which involves inserting a thin, flexible tube with a camera into the esophagus to directly observe structural problems like strictures, tumors, or inflammation.

In some cases, especially when neurological issues are suspected, doctors might recommend a videofluoroscopic swallow study (VFSS). This video X-ray technique captures the mechanics of swallowing in real-time, enabling specialists to see how food moves through the pharynx and esophagus. For evaluating the muscle activity of the esophagus, manometry can be employed. This test measures the rhythmic muscle contractions, or peristalsis, and the coordination and strength of the esophagus when swallowing.

Treatment for dysphagia is often multifaceted, depending on the underlying cause and severity. When the cause is primarily due to muscle or nerve dysfunction, speech and language therapists often lead swallowing therapy. This therapy includes exercises to strengthen the muscles, improve coordination, and learn new swallowing techniques to ensure safety. In cases of oropharyngeal dysphagia, these exercises may focus on enhancing the range of motion of the tongue and throat muscles.

Dietary modifications are also a critical part of treatment. Depending on the severity and type of dysphagia, diets may be adjusted in texture. Foods may be pureed, thickened, or prepared in a way that makes chewing and swallowing easier and safer. Nutritionists or dietitians play an important role in ensuring that individuals receive adequate nutrition from these modified diets.

For structural abnormalities like strictures or tumors, medical interventions may include dilation, where a balloon is used to stretch and widen the esophagus, or surgical procedures to remove blockages. In cases like achalasia, where the esophagus fails to relax and allow food into the stomach, options include pneumatic dilation or surgery to cut the muscle at the end of the esophagus.

Lifestyle changes are often recommended alongside medical treatments. These may include eating smaller, more frequent meals, staying upright during and after eating to prevent reflux, and avoiding foods that can irritate the esophagus or lead to additional complications. Stress management techniques and adjustments to eating habits, such as taking smaller bites and chewing thoroughly, also play a vital role in managing dysphagia effectively.

Chapter 2

Nutritional Needs for Dysphagia Management

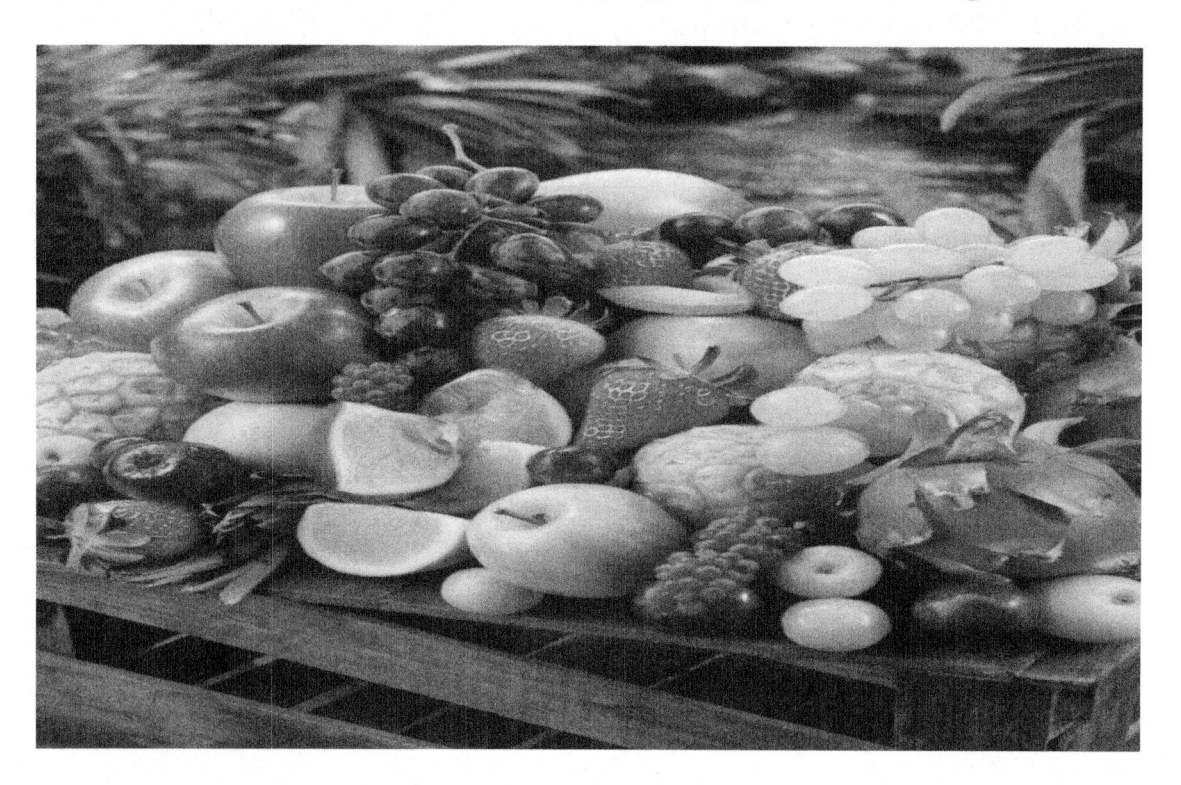

Managing dysphagia effectively involves not only modifying the texture of food to ensure safety but also carefully balancing the diet to meet nutritional needs. Proper hydration is paramount, as swallowing difficulties can often lead to decreased fluid intake, increasing the risk of dehydration. Individuals with dysphagia are encouraged to consume adequate fluids, which may need to be thickened to safer consistencies to prevent aspiration. These fluids are vital for overall health and help to facilitate the passage of food through the esophagus.

Protein is another critical component of a dysphagia-friendly diet. Adequate protein intake is essential for muscle strength and repair, which can be particularly important for those with dysphagia resulting from neurological or muscular conditions. High-protein foods like pureed meats, well-cooked legumes, or smooth cottage cheese can be incorporated into the diet. When regular food intake is challenging, protein supplements in the form of smooth shakes or blended soups might be necessary.

Fiber intake must also be carefully managed. While fiber is important for digestive health and regular bowel movements, individuals with dysphagia might find high-fiber foods difficult to swallow. Therefore, soft, cooked fruits and vegetables, well-pureed with no skins or seeds, can provide necessary fiber without compromising the safety of the diet. In some cases, a fiber supplement may be recommended if adequate levels cannot be achieved through modified diet alone.

Caloric intake is a major concern, especially for those who find eating laborious and tiring, which might lead to reduced food consumption. This can result in weight loss and malnutrition. Energy-dense foods that are easy to consume in small quantities can help maintain caloric intake. Options include smooth nut butters, avocado, and oils or cream added to purees and soups. Careful attention must be given to ensure that meals are not only safe and easy to swallow but also calorically sufficient to meet the individual's energy needs.

Overall, the diet for someone with dysphagia should be carefully planned to include all essential nutrients. Collaboration with healthcare professionals such as dietitians, speech therapists, and physicians is important to create a balanced diet that supports the individual's health while accommodating their swallowing abilities. This comprehensive approach ensures that despite the challenges of dysphagia, nutritional health is maintained, supporting better overall well-being and quality of life.

Overview of Dysphagia Diet Levels (Pureed, Mechanically Altered, Advanced)

Managing dysphagia involves adhering to specific diet levels to ensure safety and nutritional adequacy while minimizing the risk of choking and aspiration. These levels vary based on the severity of swallowing difficulties and are typically categorized into three main stages: pureed, mechanically altered, and advanced. Each stage is designed to meet the individual's needs as their ability to safely swallow different textures improves.

The pureed diet is the most restrictive and is necessary for individuals with severe dysphagia who have very limited swallowing ability. Foods in this diet are blended to a smooth, homogeneous consistency, similar to pudding or mousse, without any solid pieces. This level of diet helps prevent choking and is easier to swallow. Common foods include pureed fruits, vegetables, meats, and cooked cereals. Even liquids such as juice or milk may need to be thickened to prevent aspiration.

Moving to a slightly less restrictive diet, the **mechanically altered diet** includes foods that are soft and moist but have some cohesiveness. Foods are well-cooked and then chopped, ground, or mashed to a consistency that is easy to chew and swallow yet still has some texture. This diet is suitable for those who can manage some chewing but still need to avoid most solid foods. Examples include ground or finely diced meats, soft fruits, and well-cooked vegetables. Bread, rice, and other grains might still need to be modified or avoided depending on individual tolerance.

The **advanced diet** is less restrictive than the pureed or mechanically altered diets and is designed for individuals who are nearing a return to a regular texture diet but still need to avoid hard, sticky, or very crunchy foods. Foods in this category can be soft and tender, and require more chewing ability. Individuals on this diet might eat soft bread, rice, moist tender meats, and soft cooked vegetables. The key is that the foods are easy to chew and form into a bolus but are more similar to normal eating, providing a transition back to standard textures.

Each level of the dysphagia diet is intended to match the specific swallowing capabilities of the individual, ensuring safety while promoting the enjoyment of food and adequate nutritional intake. Modifications within each level can be tailored further by healthcare professionals to meet calorie, protein, and other nutritional needs, ensuring a comprehensive approach to managing dysphagia.

Cooking Techniques for Dysphagia

Steaming, poaching, and cooking methods for tender foods

Cooking for dysphagia involves using techniques that ensure foods are soft, moist, and easy to swallow, while still providing nutritional value and taste. Key techniques like steaming, poaching, and other gentle cooking methods are especially beneficial as they help maintain the integrity of the food's flavor, prevent drying out, and achieve the desired tenderness necessary for safe swallowing.

Steaming is one of the most effective cooking methods for preparing foods for a dysphagia diet. This technique uses the gentle heat of steam to cook foods thoroughly without direct contact with water, which can leach nutrients and flavors. Vegetables, fish, and even chicken can be steamed to a soft consistency that's easy to puree or mash. Steaming is particularly advantageous because it preserves the natural colors and nutrients of foods, making meals more appealing and nutritionally beneficial.

Poaching is another excellent method for preparing tender foods suitable for dysphagia diets. It involves cooking ingredients at a low temperature in a gently simmering liquid such as water, broth, or milk. This technique is ideal for eggs, poultry, fish, and fruits, which become soft enough to easily mash or blend while absorbing additional flavors from the poaching liquid. Poached foods are inherently moist, which helps prevent dryness that can make swallowing difficult.

Other gentle cooking methods include slow cooking and braising, which are particularly suitable for making tougher cuts of meat very tender and moist. These methods involve cooking foods slowly in a covered pot with some liquid, which breaks down tough fibers without drying out the meat, making it easier to chew and swallow for individuals with dysphagia. These techniques also enhance the flavor of the food, making meals more enjoyable.

When preparing foods for someone with dysphagia, it's important to consider not only the softness and moisture content of the food but also its overall appeal. Adding herbs and spices can improve flavor without needing to rely on texture. Furthermore, incorporating a variety of colors and aromas can make meals visually and olfactorily stimulating, which is important since mealtime enjoyment can be greatly diminished by dysphagia.

In sum, choosing the right cooking techniques is crucial for preparing meals that are safe, nutritious, and enjoyable for individuals with dysphagia. Steaming, poaching, slow cooking, and braising are all excellent methods that can be employed to create diverse, flavorful, and appropriate meals that meet the textural requirements of a dysphagia diet.

Food Texture Modification

Pureeing, thickening, and chopping techniques

Modifying the texture of food is a critical aspect of managing dysphagia to ensure safety and nutritional intake. Techniques like pureeing, thickening, and chopping are employed to make foods easier to swallow without compromising their nutritional value.

Pureeing is one of the most commonly used methods for preparing food for those with severe dysphagia. This technique involves blending foods until they reach a smooth, cohesive consistency that is similar to pudding or baby food. Almost any food can be pureed, including meats, vegetables, fruits, and grains. When pureeing, it's essential to add enough liquid, such as broth, milk, or water, to achieve the right texture. This not only helps in creating a smooth blend but also ensures that the food is moist enough to swallow easily.

Thickening is another crucial technique used for liquids rather than solids. People with dysphagia often have difficulty swallowing thin liquids, which can increase the risk of choking or aspiration. Thickening agents like commercial starch-based thickeners, gelatin, or naturally thick liquids like banana smoothies or avocado puree are used to bring liquids to a safer consistency. The thickness needed can vary from a nectar-like consistency, which is slightly thicker than water, to a honey-like consistency, which can hold its shape momentarily. Care must be taken to ensure that drinks are thickened to the recommended level for each individual's swallowing ability.

Chopping is a less intensive form of food texture modification, used for individuals who have mild to moderate dysphagia and can handle some chewing. Foods are cut into very small, uniform pieces that are easier to manage than regular-sized bites. Chopping can be adjusted to various levels, from finely chopped to ground, depending on the person's capability. This method allows for more textural variety in the diet and can be used in combination with cooking techniques such as steaming or poaching to soften the food further.

When modifying food textures for dysphagia, it's crucial to maintain a balance between safety, nutrition, and the enjoyment of food. Each modification should consider the individual's specific needs and preferences to ensure that meals are both safe to consume and satisfying. Employing these techniques effectively can greatly enhance the quality of life for those living with dysphagia, making mealtime a more pleasant and less stressful experience.

Stocking Your Pantry: Ingredients for Easy Swallowing

Stocking your pantry with the right ingredients is crucial when preparing meals for someone with dysphagia. Choosing foods that can be easily modified to meet the necessary texture requirements while still providing nutritional value and flavor is essential. Here are some staple ingredients that can help create a variety of safe and enjoyable dishes.

Liquids for Pureeing and Thickening

- **Broths and stocks**: Chicken, beef, or vegetable broths are great for pureeing meats and vegetables, adding flavor without too much salt.
- **Milk and cream**: Useful for pureeing and enriching dishes like mashed potatoes, soups, or smoothies.
- **Non-dairy alternatives**: Almond, soy, or oat milk can be used as a lactose-free option to add creaminess to pureed foods and beverages.

Protein Sources

- **Cooked meats:** Tender, cooked chicken, turkey, or beef that can be easily pureed or finely chopped.
- **Fish:** Soft fish like salmon or cod that can be steamed or poached and mashed into a suitable consistency.

- **Legumes**: Canned or cooked beans and lentils are excellent for pureeing into dips and spreads.

Starches and Grains

- **Instant cereals**: Instant oatmeal or cream of wheat that can be adjusted to a very soft consistency.
- **Soft breads**: Breads without crusts that can be soaked and made into a paste or used in bread puddings.
- **Pasta and rice**: Cooked until very soft, these can be a good base for many dishes and are easily pureed.

Fruits and Vegetables

- **Canned fruits and vegetables**: These are often softer than their fresh counterparts and can be mashed or pureed without additional cooking.
- **Avocados and bananas**: Naturally soft and creamy, perfect for mashing and require minimal preparation.
- **Applesauce and pumpkin** puree: Ready-to-use options that are smooth and can be mixed into other dishes or eaten alone.

Thickeners

- **Commercial thickeners**: Readily available thickeners that can adjust the consistency of liquids to make them safer to swallow.

- **Cornstarch and potato starch**: Natural options for thickening soups and sauces.

Seasonings and Flavor Enhancers

- Herbs and spices: Fresh or dried, these can add flavor without needing to use salt or sugar.
- Nutritional yeast: Offers a cheese-like flavor while adding vitamins, particularly B-vitamins.
- Salt and pepper: Basic seasonings that enhance the natural flavors of foods.

Miscellaneous

- Nut butters: Smooth peanut or almond butter can add protein and flavor to smoothies or desserts.
- - Honey and syrups: Can sweeten dishes if sugars need to be moderated, also useful for thickening.
- Cooking oils and butter: Essential for cooking and can add calories where needed.

Grocery shopping guide

Dairy and Dairy Alternatives

- Fullfat milk
- Cream
- Cottage cheese
- Ricotta cheese
- Almond milk
- Soy milk
- Oat milk

Proteins:

- Chicken thighs
- Beef brisket
- Pork shoulder

Fruits and Vegetables:

- Canned fruits (no sugar added)
- Canned vegetables (low sodium)
- Avocado
- Banana
- Ripe pears
- Peaches
- Squash
- Carrots
- Broccoli
- Spinach

Grains and Cereals

- Tender fish (e.g., salmon, trout, tilapia)
- Eggs
- Canned or dried beans and lentils

Healthy Fats:

- Olive oil
- canola oil)
- Avocado oil
- Butter

Seasonings

- Salt
- Pepper
- Fresh herbs (e.g., parsley, basil)
- Dried spices (e.g., cinnamon, nutmeg)

- Cream of wheat
- Grits
- Pasta
- Rice
- Instant oatmeal

Thickening Agents and Flavor Enhancers

- Commercial thickeners (e.g., starch-based thickeners)
- Cornstarch
- Potato starch
- Nut butters (e.g., smooth peanut, almond)
- Honey
- Maple syrup

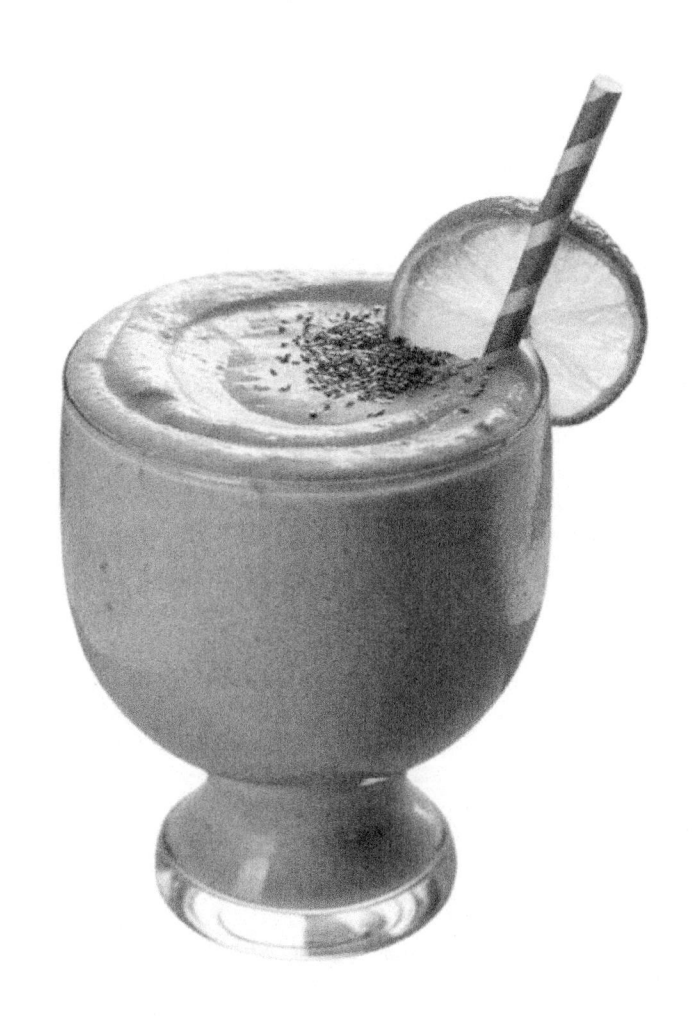

Chapter 3

Breakfast Recipes

Smoothies and Thickened Beverages

Classic Banana Smoothie

Prep Time: 5 mins | Cook Time: 0 mins | Serves: 1

Per Serving: Calories: 210 | Fat: 3g | Carbs: 45g | Fiber: 3g | Protein: 5g

Ingredients:

- 1 ripe banana

- 1 cup whole milk

- 1 tablespoon honey

- Commercial thickener as needed

Procedure:

1. Peel the banana and place it into the blender.

2. Add the cup of whole milk and the tablespoon of honey to the blender.

3. Blend all the ingredients on high until completely smooth. This should take about 1-2 minutes, ensuring no lumps remain.

4. Evaluate the consistency of the smoothie. If it needs thickening, add the commercial thickener gradually, blending after each addition, until the desired thickness is achieved.

5. Pour the smoothie into a glass and serve immediately for best taste and texture.

Blueberry Almond Smoothie

Prep Time: 5 mins | Cook Time: 0 mins | Serves: 1

Per Serving: Calories: 255 | Fat: 9g | Carbs: 38g | Fiber: 4g | Protein: 8g

Ingredients:

- 1 cup blueberries (fresh or frozen)
- 1 cup almond milk
- 2 tablespoons almond butter
- Commercial thickener as needed

Procedure:

1. Add the blueberries, almond milk, and almond butter into the blender.

2. Blend on high speed until the mixture is smooth

3. Check the consistency of your smoothie. If it is too thin for safe swallowing, gradually mix in the commercial thickener, blending well after each addition until you reach the needed thickness.

4. Once the desired thickness is reached, pour the smoothie into a glass and serve immediately.

Creamy Avocado Smoothie

Prep Time: 5 mins | Cook Time: 0 mins | Serves: 1

Per Serving: Calories: 320 | Fat: 20g | Carbs: 35g | Fiber: 7g | Protein: 4g

Ingredients:

- 1 ripe avocado

- 1 cup coconut water

- 1 teaspoon lime juice

- 1 tablespoon agave syrup or honey

- Commercial thickener as needed

Procedure:

1. Cut the avocado in half, remove the pit, and scoop the flesh into the blender.

2. Add coconut water, lime juice, and agave syrup or honey to the blender.

3. Blend all ingredients on high until the mixture is very smooth, approximately 1-2 minutes.

4. If the smoothie is too thin, gradually add commercial thickener and blend until you achieve a consistency that's easy to swallow.

5. Serve the smoothie immediately after reaching the desired thickness, ensuring it's fresh and smooth.

Peach Ginger Smoothie

Prep Time: 5 mins | Cook Time: 0 mins | Serves: 1

Per Serving: Calories: 180 | Fat: 1g | Carbs: 43g | Fiber: 2g | Protein: 2g

Ingredients:

- 1 cup sliced peaches (fresh or canned in juice)
- 1/2 teaspoon fresh grated ginger
- 1 cup apple juice
- Commercial thickener as needed

Procedure:

1. Place the sliced peaches into the blender. If using canned peaches, ensure they are drained well.
2. Add the fresh grated ginger and apple juice to the blender.
3. Blend all the ingredients on high until the mixture becomes completely smooth.
4. Assess the consistency; if the smoothie is too thin for safe swallowing, add a small amount of commercial thickener and blend again. Repeat as necessary until the desired thickness is achieved.
5. Serve the smoothie immediately, ensuring it's fresh and has the right consistency for safe swallowing.

Strawberry Coconut Smoothie

Prep Time: 5 mins | Cook Time: 0 mins | Serves: 1

Per Serving: Calories: 200 | Fat: 8g | Carbs: 30g | Fiber: 3g | Protein: 2g

Ingredients:

- 1 cup strawberries (fresh or frozen)
- 1 cup coconut milk
- 1 tablespoon honey
- Commercial thickener as needed

Procedure:

1. Add the strawberries and coconut milk to the blender.
2. Pour in the tablespoon of honey for a natural sweetener.
3. Blend on high until the ingredients are fully combined and the texture is smooth
4. Check the thickness of the smoothie. If required, gradually incorporate commercial thickener, blending after each addition until it meets the swallowing needs.
5. Once the smoothie is properly thickened, pour into a glass and serve promptly.

Mango Lassi Smoothie

Prep Time: 5 mins | Cook Time: 0 mins | Serves: 1

Per Serving: Calories: 210 | Fat: 3g | Carbs: 42g | Fiber: 2g | Protein: 6g

Ingredients:

- 1 cup mango chunks (fresh or frozen)
- 1/2 cup plain yogurt
- 1/2 cup water
- 1 tablespoon honey
- Commercial thickener as needed

Procedure:

1. Combine the mango chunks, plain yogurt, water, and honey in the blender.

2. Blend until smooth

3. If the smoothie's texture is too fluid, slowly mix in the thickener, blending thoroughly after each addition until you achieve the necessary consistency.

4. Serve the mango lassi smoothie immediately after it reaches the perfect thickness, ensuring it is fresh and enjoyable.

You might be wondering why I include Commercial Thickeners in the recipes.

Including commercial thickeners in smoothie recipes for dysphagia patients is crucial for several reasons. They ensure safety by reducing the risk of choking and aspiration, allow for precise consistency adjustments to meet individual swallowing needs, and maintain the original flavor of beverages. Thickeners are easy to use, making meal preparation simpler and ensuring that patients can safely consume a variety of nutritious drinks. This helps prevent nutritional deficiencies and dehydration, which are common challenges for those with dysphagia.

Soft Pancakes and Modified Eggs

Classic Soft Pancakes

Prep Time: 5 mins | Cook Time: 10 mins | Serves: 2

Ingredients:

- 1 cup pancake mix
- 3/4 cup whole milk
- 1 egg
- Butter for cooking

Procedure:

1. Blend the batter: In a blender, combine the pancake mix, whole milk, and egg. Blend until the mixture is completely smooth, ensuring there are no lumps.

2. Preheat the skillet: Place a non-stick skillet over medium heat on the stove. Add a small amount of butter and allow it to melt, spreading it around to coat the surface of the skillet.

3. Cook the pancakes: Pour small ladles of batter onto the hot skillet. Cook the first side until bubbles form on the surface and the edges appear set, about 2-3 minutes. Use a spatula to gently flip each pancake and cook the other side until golden brown, another 2-3 minutes.

4. Remove the pancakes from the skillet and place them on a plate. Serve warm with toppings of your choice, such as pureed fruit or syrup, suitable for dysphagia diets.

Silken Scrambled Eggs

Prep Time: 2 mins | Cook Time: 5 mins | Serves: 1

Ingredients:

- 2 eggs
- 1/4 cup milk
- Salt to taste
- Butter for cooking

Procedure:

1. Mix the eggs: In a mixing bowl, whisk together the eggs and milk until well combined and smooth. Add a pinch of salt to taste.

2. Cook the eggs: Heat a non-stick skillet over low heat. Add a small amount of butter, letting it melt. Pour in the egg mixture. Cook slowly, stirring gently and constantly with a rubber spatula. This helps prevent the eggs from sticking to the pan and ensures they stay soft and creamy.

3. Monitor the texture: Keep the heat low and continue to stir. Remove the pan from the heat when the eggs are mostly set but still slightly runny. They will continue to cook from the residual heat, reaching the perfect consistency.

4. Serve the eggs right away while they are warm and soft, ensuring they are easy to swallow.

Oatmeal Banana Pancakes

Prep Time: 10 mins | Cook Time: 10 mins | Serves: 2

Ingredients:

- 1 ripe banana, mashed
- 1/2 cup cooked oatmeal
- 1 egg
- 1/4 cup milk
- 1/2 cup all-purpose flour

Procedure:

1. Mix the wet ingredients: In a bowl, combine the mashed banana, cooked oatmeal, egg, and milk. Stir well until all the ingredients are fully blended.

2. Add dry ingredients: Gradually mix in the flour until the batter is smooth and without lumps.

3. Cook the pancakes: Heat a non-stick skillet over medium heat and lightly grease it with butter or oil. Pour small amounts of batter onto the skillet, cooking for about 3-4 minutes on each side until the pancakes are golden brown and cooked through.

4. Serve: These pancakes are soft and easy to swallow. Serve warm with a dollop of yogurt or a drizzle of honey if desired.

Soft Poached Eggs

Prep Time: 2 mins | Cook Time: 3 mins | Serves: 1

Ingredients:

- 1 egg
- Water for poaching
- Salt to taste

Procedure:

1. Prepare the water: Fill a small saucepan with water and bring it to a gentle simmer. Add a pinch of salt.

2. Poach the egg: Crack the egg into a small cup or bowl. Gently slide the egg from the cup into the simmering water. Cook for about 3 minutes until the egg white is set but the yolk remains soft.

3. Remove and serve: Using a slotted spoon, carefully lift the egg out of the water. Serve immediately, ensuring it's soft enough to be easily swallowed. This method keeps the egg moist and easy to consume.

Pumpkin Spice Pancakes

Prep Time: 10 mins | Cook Time: 10 mins | Serves: 2

Ingredients:

- 1/2 cup pumpkin puree

- 1 cup all-purpose flour

- 1 egg

- 3/4 cup milk

- 1 teaspoon pumpkin pie spice

- 1 tablespoon sugar

- Butter for cooking

Procedure:

1. Combine the ingredients: In a large bowl, mix the pumpkin puree, egg, and milk until smooth. Add the flour, pumpkin pie spice, and sugar, and stir until just combined; avoid overmixing to keep the pancakes tender.

2. Cook the pancakes: Heat a non-stick skillet over medium heat and lightly grease it with butter. Pour small amounts of batter onto the skillet. Cook until bubbles appear

on the surface, about 3-4 minutes, then flip and cook for an additional 2-3 minutes until golden and fluffy.

3. These pancakes are soft and carry the comforting flavor of pumpkin spice. Serve with a drizzle of maple syrup or a dollop of whipped cream for extra indulgence.

Creamy Baked Eggs

Prep Time: 5 mins | Cook Time: 15 mins | Serves: 2

Ingredients:

- 4 eggs
- 1/4 cup cream
- Salt and pepper to taste
- Butter for greasing

Procedure:

1. Preheat the oven and prepare dishes: Preheat your oven to 350°F (175°C). Grease two small baking dishes with butter.

2. Add eggs and cream: Crack two eggs into each dish. Pour two tablespoons of cream over each set of eggs and season with salt and pepper.

3. Bake the eggs: Place the dishes in the oven and bake for about 15 minutes, or until the egg whites are set but the yolks are still runny.

4. These eggs will be creamy and soft, ideal for easy swallowing. Serve immediately, perhaps with a side of soft toast that has been lightly buttered and cut into small, manageable pieces.

Apple Cinnamon Pancakes

Prep Time: 10 mins | Cook Time: 10 mins | Serves: 2

Ingredients:

- 1/2 cup finely grated apple
- 1 cup all-purpose flour
- 1 egg
- 3/4 cup milk
- 1 teaspoon cinnamon
- 1 tablespoon sugar
- Butter for cooking

Procedure:

1. Prepare the batter: In a large mixing bowl, combine the grated apple, egg, and milk. Stir until well mixed. Add flour, cinnamon, and sugar to the apple mixture and stir until just combined.

2. Cook the pancakes: Heat a non-stick skillet over medium heat and add a small amount of butter to coat the surface. Pour scoops of batter onto the skillet, cooking

until bubbles form on the surface and the edges look set, about 3-4 minutes. Flip the pancakes and cook for another 2-3 minutes on the other side.

3. Serve these moist, flavor-rich pancakes with a soft topping like applesauce or yogurt, perfect for an easy-to-swallow breakfast or snack.

Egg and Avocado Mash

Prep Time: 5 mins | Cook Time: 5 mins | Serves: 1

Ingredients:

- 1 ripe avocado
- 2 eggs
- Salt and pepper to taste

Procedure:

1. Cook the eggs: In a skillet, scramble the eggs over low heat, stirring frequently, until they are just set but still very moist.

2. Prepare the avocado: While the eggs are cooking, peel and mash the avocado in a bowl until smooth.

3. Combine and serve: Mix the scrambled eggs into the mashed avocado. Season with salt and pepper to taste. This combination creates a creamy, easy-to-swallow dish packed with nutrients.

Nutritious Porridges and Cereals

Classic Oatmeal Porridge

Prep Time: 5 mins | Cook Time: 10 mins | Serves: 1

Ingredients:

- 1/2 cup rolled oats
- 1 cup milk or water
- 1 tablespoon honey
- 1/2 teaspoon cinnamon

Procedure:

1. In a small pot, combine rolled oats and milk or water. Bring to a simmer over medium heat.

2. Reduce heat and cook, stirring frequently, until the oats are very soft and the porridge has thickened, about 10 minutes.

3. Stir in honey and cinnamon before serving. Blend to a smooth consistency if necessary for easier swallowing.

Creamy Rice Pudding

Prep Time: 5 mins | Cook Time: 30 mins | Serves: 2

Ingredients:

- 1/2 cup short-grain rice
- 2 cups milk
- 2 tablespoons sugar
- 1 teaspoon vanilla extract

Procedure:

1. Combine rice and milk in a saucepan. Bring to a boil, then reduce heat to low.

2. Simmer gently, stirring occasionally, until the rice is very soft and the mixture has thickened, about 30 minutes.

3. Stir in sugar and vanilla extract. Blend the pudding to achieve a smooth texture for safer swallowing.

Polenta Porridge

Prep Time: 5 mins | Cook Time: 20 mins | Serves: 1

Ingredients:

- 1/4 cup polenta

- 1 cup water or broth of your choice (vegetable or meat)

- 1 tablespoon grated cheese

- 1 teaspoon butter

Procedure:

1. In a saucepan, bring water or broth to a boil. Gradually stir in polenta.

2. Reduce heat to low and cook, stirring often, until the mixture is thick and the polenta grains are soft, about 20 minutes.

3. Add grated cheese and butter, stirring until melted and fully incorporated. Blend if necessary to achieve a smooth texture.

Barley Porridge

Prep Time: 5 mins | Cook Time: 25 mins | Serves: 1

Ingredients:

- 1/4 cup hulled barley
- 1 cup water or milk
- 1 tablespoon maple syrup
- Pinch of salt

Procedure:

1. Rinse barley thoroughly under cold water.

2. In a saucepan, combine barley and water or milk. Bring to a boil, then reduce heat to a low simmer.

3. Cook, covered, stirring occasionally, until the barley is very soft and the mixture has a thick consistency, about 25 minutes.

4. Stir in maple syrup and a pinch of salt. Blend the porridge to a smooth texture if necessary before serving.

Quinoa Breakfast Porridge

Prep Time: 5 mins | Cook Time: 15 mins | Serves: 1

Ingredients:

- 1/4 cup quinoa, rinsed

- 1 cup almond milk

- 1 tablespoon honey

- 1/4 teaspoon cinnamon

Procedure:

1. In a pot, combine rinsed quinoa and almond milk. Bring to a boil.

2. Reduce heat to low and simmer, covered, until the quinoa is tender and the porridge is creamy, about 15 minutes.

3. Stir in honey and cinnamon. For a smoother consistency, blend the porridge before serving.

Millet Porridge

Prep Time: 5 mins | Cook Time: 20 mins | Serves: 1

Ingredients:

- 1/4 cup millet

- 1 cup coconut milk

- 1 tablespoon agave syrup

- Procedure:

1. Toast millet in a dry saucepan over medium heat for 3-4 minutes until slightly golden.

2. Add coconut milk and bring to a boil. Reduce heat and simmer, covered, until millet is tender and the porridge is thick, about 20 minutes.

3. Stir in agave syrup. Blend the porridge for a smoother consistency if preferred.

Buckwheat Porridge

Prep Time: 5 mins | Cook Time: 10 mins | Serves: 1

Ingredients:

- 1/4 cup buckwheat groats
- 1 cup water
- 1 tablespoon brown sugar
- 1/4 teaspoon vanilla extract

Procedure:

1. Rinse buckwheat groats under cold water until water runs clear.

2. In a saucepan, combine buckwheat and water. Bring to a boil, then reduce heat and simmer until soft and thickened, about 10 minutes.

3. Stir in brown sugar and vanilla extract. For those who require a very smooth texture, blend the porridge to desired consistency.

Sweet Potato and Rice Porridge

Prep Time: 10 mins | Cook Time: 25 mins | Serves: 1

Ingredients:

- 1/4 cup finely grated sweet potato

- 1/4 cup rice

- 1 cup milk

- 1 tablespoon maple syrup

Procedure:

1. Combine sweet potato, rice, and milk in a saucepan. Bring to a simmer over medium heat.

2. Reduce heat to low and cook, stirring occasionally, until the rice is completely soft and the porridge is thick, about 25 minutes.

3. Stir in maple syrup. Blend to a smooth consistency for easier swallowing.

Apple and Cinnamon Buckwheat Porridge

Prep Time: 5 mins | Cook Time: 10 mins | Serves: 1

Ingredients:

- 1/4 cup buckwheat groats
- 1 small apple, peeled and finely grated
- 1 cup water
- 1/2 teaspoon cinnamon
- 1 tablespoon honey

Procedure:

1. Rinse buckwheat under cold water. In a saucepan, combine buckwheat, grated apple, and water. Bring to a boil.

2. Reduce heat and simmer until the buckwheat is tender and the porridge has thickened, about 10 minutes.

3. Stir in cinnamon and honey. Blend the porridge if a smoother texture is required.

Chapter 4: Soups and Stews

Hearty Vegetable Soup

Before we begins with the vegetable soup I want you to make your Broth first because this is needed for most of the recipes

Making broth is a fundamental cooking skill that can enhance the flavor of many dishes. Broths can be made from vegetables, meat, or a combination of both.

Making vegetable broth is a simple and rewarding process that allows you to utilize leftover vegetables and scraps, transforming them into a flavorful base for soups, stews, and other dishes.

Vegetable Broth

Ingredients:

- 2 onions, chopped

- 2 carrots, chopped

- 3 celery stalks, chopped

- 1 garlic clove, smashed (optional)

- 1 bay leaf

- A few sprigs of thyme or parsley

- Salt and pepper to taste

- Water

Procedure:

1. Prepare Vegetables: Chop your vegetables into large chunks. You can also include other vegetables like mushrooms, leeks, or tomatoes for more depth of flavor.

2. Cook Vegetables: In a large pot, add a little oil and sauté the onions, carrots, and celery until they start to soften. Add garlic if using.

3. Add Water and Simmer: Cover the vegetables with water. Bring to a boil and then reduce to a simmer.

4. Add Herbs and Seasonings: Add the bay leaf, thyme, parsley, and a good pinch of salt and pepper.

5. Simmer: Let the broth simmer uncovered for at least 1 hour. The longer it simmers, the more flavorful it will be.

6. Strain and Store: Strain the broth through a fine-mesh sieve, discarding the solids. Adjust the seasoning if necessary. Store in the refrigerator for up to a week or freeze for longer storage.

Chicken or Beef Broth

Ingredients:

- Bones from chicken or beef
- 1 onion, chopped
- 1 carrot, chopped
- 1 celery stalk, chopped
- 1 bay leaf

- Water

Procedure:

1. Roast Bones (optional but recommended for depth of flavor): Place the bones on a baking sheet and roast at 400°F (200°C) until golden, about 30 minutes.

2. Prepare the Pot: Place the roasted bones in a large pot. Add the chopped vegetables and bay leaf.

3. Cover with Water: Fill the pot with water until the bones and vegetables are fully submerged.

4. Simmer: Bring to a boil, then reduce the heat and simmer gently for 3-4 hours for chicken bones or 6-8 hours for beef bones. Skim off any foam or impurities that rise to the surface.

5. Strain and Store: Strain the broth through a fine-mesh sieve. Discard the solids. Store the broth in the refrigerator or freeze for future use.

These simple methods will give you a flavorful base for soups, sauces, gravies, and other dishes. Making broth at home not only ensures that you can control the ingredients and avoid preservatives but also allows you to make use of scraps that might otherwise be wasted.

Now let's begin !

Creamy Carrot Soup

Prep Time: 10 mins | Cook Time: 20 mins | Serves: 2

Per Serving: Calories: 180 | Fat: 9g | Carbs: 22g | Fiber: 5g | Protein: 3g

Ingredients:

- 4 large carrots, peeled and chopped
- 1 small onion, chopped
- 2 cups vegetable broth
- 1 teaspoon grated ginger
- 1/4 cup cream

Procedure:

1. In a pot, sauté onions and ginger until soft.
2. Add chopped carrots and vegetable broth. Bring to a boil, then simmer until carrots are very soft, about 20 minutes.
3. Blend the mixture until completely smooth.
4. Return soup to the pot, stir in cream, heat through, and adjust seasoning.

Butternut Squash Soup

Prep Time: 15 mins | Cook Time: 30 mins | Serves: 2

Per Serving: Calories: 175 | Fat: 3g | Carbs: 37g | Fiber: 6g | Protein: 3g

- Ingredients:

- 1/2 butternut squash, peeled and cubed
- 1 onion, chopped
- 2 cups vegetable broth
- 1/4 teaspoon nutmeg

Procedure:

1. On a baking sheet, roast the butternut squash and onion at 375°F until tender, about 25 minutes.

2. Transfer the roasted vegetables to a pot, add vegetable broth, and simmer for 5 minutes.

3. Puree the soup until smooth, stir in nutmeg, and heat through.

Broccoli and Cheddar Soup

Prep Time: 10 mins | Cook Time: 20 mins | Serves: 2

Per Serving: Calories: 250 | Fat: 16g | Carbs: 15g | Fiber: 4g | Protein: 12g

Ingredients:

- 2 cups broccoli florets

- 1 small onion, chopped

- 1 cup vegetable broth

- 1/2 cup cheddar cheese, shredded

- 1/2 cup cream

Procedure:

1. In a pot, sauté onion until soft.

2. Add broccoli and broth, simmer until broccoli is very tender, about 15 minutes.

3. Blend the soup to a smooth texture.

4. Return to the pot, add cheese and cream, stir until cheese melts and soup is heated through.

Potato Leek Soup

Prep Time: 10 mins | Cook Time: 25 mins | Serves: 2

Per Serving: Calories: 220 | Fat: 8g | Carbs: 34g | Fiber: 3g | Protein: 4g

Ingredients:

- 2 large potatoes, peeled and diced

- 1 leek, cleaned and sliced

- 2 cups vegetable broth

- 1/4 cup cream

- Salt and pepper to taste

Procedure:

1. In a pot, sauté leeks in a little oil until soft.

2. Add diced potatoes and vegetable broth, bring to a boil, then simmer until potatoes are very tender, about 20 minutes.

3. Blend the mixture until completely smooth.

4. Stir in cream, season with salt and pepper, and heat through before serving.

Tomato Basil Soup

Prep Time: 10 mins | Cook Time: 20 mins | Serves: 2

Per Serving: Calories: 140 | Fat: 6g | Carbs: 20g | Fiber: 3g | Protein: 3g

Ingredients:

- 4 ripe tomatoes, chopped
- 1 onion, chopped
- 2 cloves garlic, minced
- 1 cup vegetable broth
- 1/4 cup fresh basil leaves
- 2 tablespoons olive oil
- Salt and pepper to taste

Procedure:

1. In a pot, heat olive oil over medium heat. Add onion and garlic, and sauté until translucent.

2. Add chopped tomatoes and vegetable broth, simmer for about 15 minutes until the tomatoes are very soft.

3. Add basil leaves, then blend the soup until smooth.

4. Season with salt and pepper, heat through, and serve warm.

Spinach and Yogurt Soup

Prep Time: 10 mins | Cook Time: 15 mins | Serves: 2

Per Serving: Calories: 150 | Fat: 6g | Carbs: 18g | Fiber: 4g | Protein: 8g

Ingredients:

- 2 cups fresh spinach

- 1 onion, chopped

- 1 cup vegetable broth

- 1/2 cup plain yogurt

- 1 tablespoon olive oil

- Salt and nutmeg to taste

Procedure:

1. In a pot, heat olive oil and sauté onion until soft.

2. Add spinach and broth, cover and simmer until the spinach is wilted, about 5 minutes.

3. Remove from heat, blend until smooth.

4. Stir in yogurt, season with salt and a pinch of nutmeg, and gently heat through without boiling.

Smooth Cream Soups

Cream of Mushroom Soup

Prep Time: 10 mins | Cook Time: 20 mins | Serves: 2

Per Serving: Calories: 180 | Fat: 14g | Carbs: 12g | Fiber: 2g | Protein: 3g

Ingredients:

- 1 cup chopped mushrooms
- 1 small onion, chopped
- 2 cups vegetable broth
- 1/2 cup heavy cream (use any store-bought pasteurized heavy cream, which is also known as whipping cream)

Procedure:

1. In a medium saucepan, cook the chopped onions and mushrooms over medium heat until they are soft and lightly browned.

2. Add the vegetable broth to the saucepan and bring to a boil. Then reduce the heat and simmer for about 15 minutes.

3. Use a blender or immersion blender or any blender you have to puree the soup until it is completely smooth.

4. Return the pureed soup to the saucepan, stir in the heavy cream, and warm it on low heat until it's hot enough to serve.

Creamy Tomato Basil Soup

Prep Time: 10 mins | Cook Time: 25 mins | Serves: 2

Per Serving: Calories: 200 | Fat: 15g | Carbs: 15g | Fiber: 3g | Protein: 3g

Ingredients:

- 4 ripe tomatoes, chopped
- 2 cloves garlic, minced
- 1/4 cup fresh basil, chopped
- 2 cups vegetable broth
- 1/2 cup heavy cream (as above, use pasteurized heavy cream suitable for cooking)

Procedure:

1. In a large pot, add the chopped tomatoes, minced garlic, and chopped basil. Pour in the vegetable broth and bring the mixture to a simmer.
2. Let the soup simmer gently for about 20 minutes or until the tomatoes are very soft.
3. Blend the soup until smooth using a blender or immersion blender.
4. Return the smooth soup to the pot, stir in the heavy cream, and heat it through on low heat. Avoid boiling after adding cream to keep the soup smooth and creamy.

Cream of Broccoli Soup

Prep Time: 10 mins | Cook Time: 20 mins | Serves: 2

Per Serving: Calories: 190 | Fat: 15g | Carbs: 11g | Fiber: 3g | Protein: 5g

Ingredients:

- 2 cups broccoli florets

- 1 small onion, chopped

- 2 cups vegetable broth

- 1/2 cup heavy cream (again, any standard pasteurized heavy cream will work)

Procedure:

1. Place the broccoli florets and chopped onion in a large pot. Add the vegetable broth and bring to a simmer.

2. Cook the broccoli and onions until they are very tender, about 15-20 minutes.

3. Blend the mixture until smooth with a blender or immersion blender.

4. Return the soup to the pot, mix in the heavy cream, and gently heat until it's ready to serve.

Cream of Asparagus Soup

Prep Time: 10 mins | Cook Time: 20 mins | Serves: 2

Per Serving: Calories: 175 | Fat: 12g | Carbs: 14g | Fiber: 3g | Protein: 4g

Ingredients:

- 1 bunch asparagus, woody ends trimmed and chopped
- 1 small onion, chopped
- 2 cups vegetable broth
- 1/2 cup heavy cream (pasteurized for cooking)

Procedure:

1. In a large pot, sauté the chopped asparagus and onion until the onion is translucent and the asparagus is slightly tender.

2. Add the vegetable broth and bring to a boil. Reduce heat and simmer until the asparagus is very soft, about 15 minutes.

3. Blend the soup using a blender or immersion blender until it is completely smooth.

4. Return the pureed soup to the pot, stir in the heavy cream, and heat on low until just hot. Serve warm.

Cream of Sweet Potato Soup

Prep Time: 15 mins | Cook Time: 25 mins | Serves: 2

Per Serving: Calories: 220 | Fat: 14g | Carbs: 24g | Fiber: 4g | Protein: 3g

Ingredients:

- 2 large sweet potatoes, peeled and cubed

- 1 small onion, chopped

- 2 cups vegetable broth

- 1/2 teaspoon ground cinnamon

- 1/2 cup heavy cream

Procedure:

1. In a pot, combine the sweet potatoes, onion, and vegetable broth. Bring to a boil, then reduce heat and simmer until the sweet potatoes are very soft, about 20 minutes.

2. Add cinnamon to the pot and stir well.

3. Blend the soup until smooth.

4. Return the soup to the pot, mix in the heavy cream, and gently warm the soup. Be sure not to boil after adding cream to maintain a smooth texture. Serve warm.

Creamy Pea Soup

Prep Time: 10 mins | Cook Time: 15 mins | Serves: 2

Per Serving: Calories: 160 | Fat: 8g | Carbs: 18g | Fiber: 5g | Protein: 6g

Ingredients:

- 2 cups frozen green peas
- 1 small onion, chopped
- 2 cups vegetable broth
- 1/2 cup heavy cream
- Fresh mint leaves for flavor (optional)

Procedure:

1. In a saucepan, sauté the onion until it's soft.
2. Add the green peas and vegetable broth, and bring to a simmer. Cook until the peas are tender, about 10 minutes.
3. Add a few fresh mint leaves if using, then blend the mixture until smooth.
4. Stir in the heavy cream and heat through on low heat, ensuring the soup does not boil.

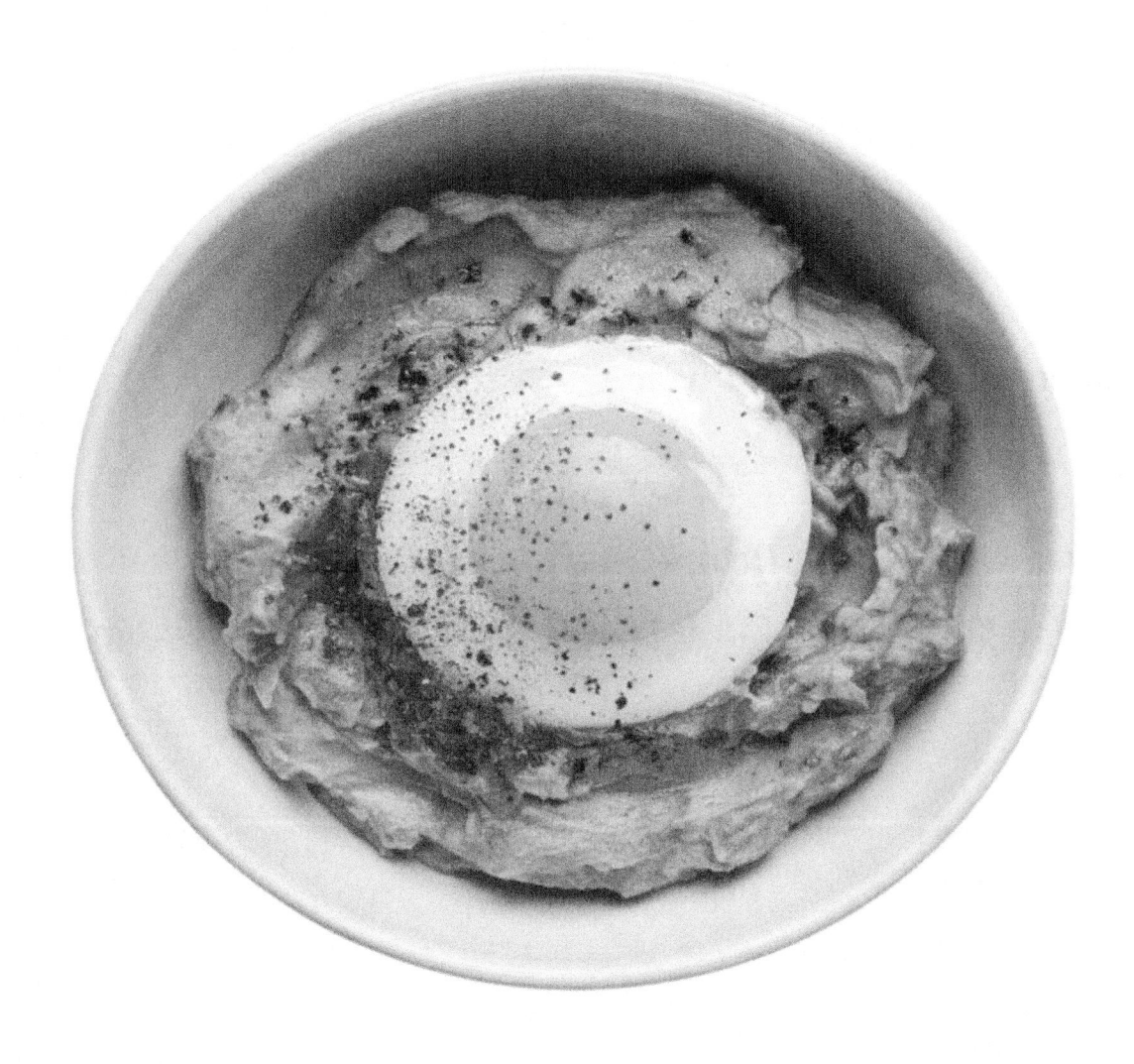

Chapter 5: Main Dishes

Protein-Rich Purees

Chicken and Vegetable Puree

Prep Time: 10 mins | Cook Time: 30 mins | Serves: 2

Per Serving: Calories: 150 | Fat: 4g | Carbs: 10g | Fiber: 2g | Protein: 20g

Ingredients:

- 1 chicken breast, boneless and skinless
- 2 large carrots, peeled
- 1/2 cup low-sodium chicken broth

Procedure:

1. Cook the Chicken: Place the chicken breast in a pot and cover with water. Bring to a boil, then reduce heat and simmer for 20 minutes or until the chicken is fully cooked and tender.

2. Steam the Carrots: While the chicken cooks, cut the carrots into rounds and steam them until they are very soft, about 15-20 minutes.

3. Blend: Place the cooked chicken and steamed carrots in a blender. Add a small amount of chicken broth and blend on high until smooth. Gradually add more broth as needed to achieve a creamy consistency.

4. Taste the puree and add a pinch of salt if needed. Ensure the texture is smooth and easy to swallow. Serve warm.

Salmon Puree

Prep Time: 5 mins | Cook Time: 15 mins | Serves: 2
Per Serving: Calories: 200 | Fat: 12g | Carbs: 1g | Fiber: 0g | Protein: 22g

Ingredients:

- 1 salmon fillet
- 2 tablespoons olive oil
- 1/4 cup water or as needed

Procedure:

1. Poach the Salmon: In a skillet, place the salmon and just enough water to cover the bottom. Cover and cook over medium heat for about 10-12 minutes, or until the salmon is cooked through and flakes easily.

2. Blend: Transfer the cooked salmon to a blender. Add olive oil and a small amount of the cooking liquid. Blend on high until smooth, adding more liquid as needed to reach a creamy consistency.

3. Check Consistency and Serve: The puree should be smooth with no lumps. Serve warm, ensuring it's soft enough for easy swallowing.

Lentil and Carrot Puree

Prep Time: 10 mins | Cook Time: 25 mins | Serves: 2

Per Serving: Calories: 180 | Fat: 5g | Carbs: 25g | Fiber: 8g | Protein: 10g

Ingredients:

- 1 cup red lentils, rinsed
- 2 large carrots, peeled and chopped
- 1/2 cup water or vegetable broth

Procedure:

1. Cook the Lentils and Carrots: In a medium pot, combine the lentils, carrots, and enough water or broth to cover. Bring to a boil, then reduce heat and simmer for about 20 minutes or until both the lentils and carrots are very soft.

2. Blend: Drain any excess liquid and transfer the mixture to a blender. Add a bit of fresh water or broth and blend until completely smooth, adding more liquid as needed to achieve a creamy texture.

3. Adjust the seasoning with a little salt if desired. Ensure the puree is perfectly smooth to make swallowing easier. Serve warm.

White Fish Puree

Prep Time: 5 mins | Cook Time: 10 mins | Serves: 2
Per Serving: Calories: 120 | Fat: 2g | Carbs: 5g | Fiber: 1g | Protein: 20g

Ingredients:

- 1 white fish fillet (e.g., cod or tilapia)
- 1/4 cup low-sodium vegetable broth
- 1 tablespoon olive oil

Procedure:

1. Cook the Fish: Place the fish fillet in a skillet over medium heat. Add just enough vegetable broth to cover the bottom of the skillet. Cover and let it steam until the fish is cooked through and flakes easily, about 8-10 minutes.

2. Blend: Transfer the cooked fish to a blender. Add olive oil and a splash of the cooking broth. Blend on high until smooth, adding more broth as needed to reach a creamy consistency.

3. Ensure the puree is lump-free and silky. If needed, pass through a sieve to remove any remaining bits. Serve warm, seasoned lightly with salt.

Black Bean Puree

Prep Time: 5 mins | Cook Time: 10 mins | Serves: 2
Per Serving: Calories: 150 | Fat: 4g | Carbs: 20g | Fiber: 8g | Protein: 8g

Ingredients:

- 1 cup cooked black beans
- 1/4 cup water or vegetable broth
- 1 teaspoon cumin
- 1 tablespoon olive oil

Procedure:

1. Prepare the Beans: If using canned black beans, rinse them thoroughly under cold water. If from dry, make sure they are cooked until very soft.

2. Blend: Put the black beans in a blender along with water or broth, cumin, and olive oil. Blend on high until completely smooth, adding more liquid if necessary to achieve a creamy consistency.

3. Taste the puree and adjust seasoning as needed. Serve warm, ensuring it's smooth enough for easy swallowing.

Turkey and Sweet Potato Puree

Prep Time: 10 mins | Cook Time: 30 mins | Serves: 2

Per Serving: Calories: 175 | Fat: 4g | Carbs: 20g | Fiber: 3g | Protein: 15g

Ingredients:

- 1 small turkey breast
- 1 medium sweet potato, peeled and cubed
- 1/2 cup low-sodium chicken broth

Procedure:

1. Cook the Turkey and Sweet Potato: In a medium pot, add the turkey breast and sweet potato cubes. Cover with water and bring to a boil. Reduce heat and simmer until both the turkey and sweet potato are very tender, about 20-25 minutes.

2. Blend: Drain the water and transfer the turkey and sweet potato to a blender. Add chicken broth and blend until smooth, adding more broth as needed for a creamy texture.

3. Adjust the salt to taste and ensure the puree is perfectly smooth for easy swallowing. Serve warm.

Tuna and Avocado Puree

Prep Time: 5 mins | Cook Time: 0 mins | Serves: 2

Per Serving: Calories: 190 | Fat: 10g | Carbs: 6g | Fiber: 4g | Protein: 20g

Ingredients:

- 1 can of tuna, drained
- 1 ripe avocado
- 1 tablespoon lemon juice
- Salt to taste

Procedure:

1. Prepare the Ingredients: Ensure the tuna is thoroughly drained. Halve the avocado, remove the pit, and scoop out the flesh.

2. Blend: Place the tuna, avocado flesh, and lemon juice in a blender. Blend until smooth, adding a splash of water if necessary to achieve a creamy consistency.

3. Season with a little salt to enhance the flavors. Serve the puree chilled, ensuring it is smooth and homogeneous for easy swallowing.

Chickpea and Olive Oil Puree

Prep Time: 5 mins | Cook Time: 0 mins | Serves: 2 Per Serving: Calories: 160 | Fat: 8g | Carbs: 18g | Fiber: 5g | Protein: 6g

Ingredients:

- 1 cup cooked chickpeas
- 2 tablespoons olive oil
- 1/4 cup water, or as needed
- 1/2 teaspoon cumin

Procedure:

1. Prepare the Chickpeas: If using canned chickpeas, rinse them well under cold water to remove excess sodium.

2. Blend: Add chickpeas, olive oil, and cumin to a blender. Start blending, gradually adding water until the mixture is completely smooth.

3. Check the consistency, ensuring it's perfectly smooth and free of lumps. Add more water if necessary to achieve a creamy texture. Serve the puree at room temperature or slightly warmed.

Beef and Potato Puree

Prep Time: 10 mins | Cook Time: 30 mins | Serves: 2

Per Serving: Calories: 220 | Fat: 9g | Carbs: 20g | Fiber: 2g | Protein: 15g

Ingredients:

- 1/2 pound lean ground beef

- 1 large potato, peeled and cubed

- 1/2 cup beef broth

Procedure:

1. Cook the Beef and Potato: In a medium pot, brown the ground beef over medium heat until fully cooked. Add the cubed potato and beef broth, bring to a boil, then reduce heat and simmer until the potato is tender, about 20 minutes.

2. Blend: Drain any excess fat and transfer the beef and potato to a blender. Blend until smooth, adding extra broth if necessary to facilitate blending.

3. Season with a pinch of salt. Ensure the puree is smooth and easy to swallow. Serve warm, adjusted for consistency to meet swallowing needs.

Soft Cooked Meat and Vegetable Combinations

Chicken and Carrot Puree

Prep Time: 10 mins | Cook Time: 25 mins | Serves: 2

Per Serving: Calories: 150 | Fat: 3g | Carbs: 10g | Fiber: 2g | Protein: 20g

Ingredients:

- 1 chicken breast
- 2 large carrots, peeled
- 1/2 cup low-sodium chicken broth

Procedure:

1. Cook the Chicken and Carrots: Place the chicken breast and peeled carrots in a medium pot. Cover with water and bring to a boil over high heat. Once boiling, reduce the heat to a simmer and cover the pot. Let it cook until the chicken is thoroughly cooked and the carrots are tender, about 20-25 minutes.

2. Blend the Ingredients: Remove the chicken and carrots from the pot and place them in a blender. Add about 1/2 cup of chicken broth to start.

3. Puree the Mixture: Blend the chicken and carrots on high until you achieve a smooth, creamy consistency. If the puree is too thick, add more broth a little at a time until you reach the desired consistency.

4. Season and Serve: Taste the puree and add a pinch of salt if needed. Serve the puree warm, ensuring it is smooth and easy to swallow.

Beef and Sweet Potato Mash

Prep Time: 15 mins | Cook Time: 30 mins | Serves: 2
Per Serving: Calories: 220 | Fat: 8g | Carbs: 20g | Fiber: 3g | Protein: 15g

Ingredients:

- 1/2 pound lean ground beef
- 1 large sweet potato, peeled and cubed
- 1/2 cup beef broth

Procedure:

1. Prepare the Beef: In a skillet over medium heat, cook the ground beef. Stir occasionally to break up the meat into small pieces. Cook until the beef is browned and no longer pink, about 8-10 minutes. Drain any excess fat.

2. Cook the Sweet Potato: While the beef is cooking, place the cubed sweet potato in a pot and cover with water. Bring to a boil and then reduce to a simmer. Cook until the sweet potatoes are very soft, about 15-20 minutes.

3. Blend Together: Drain the sweet potatoes and add them to the blender along with the cooked beef. Pour in the beef broth and blend until smooth. Add more broth if needed to achieve a creamy consistency.

4. Adjust the seasoning, adding a little salt if necessary. Ensure the texture is suitable for easy swallowing. Serve the mash warm.

Salmon and Pea Puree

Prep Time: 5 mins | Cook Time: 20 mins | Serves: 2
Per Serving: Calories: 200 | Fat: 12g | Carbs: 5g | Fiber: 2g | Protein: 18g

Ingredients:

- 1 salmon fillet
- 1 cup green peas, fresh or frozen
- 1/4 cup water or fish broth
- 1 tablespoon olive oil

Procedure:

1. Cook the Salmon: Place the salmon fillet in a skillet or baking dish. If using a skillet, add just enough water to cover the bottom of the pan, cover with a lid, and let it simmer gently for about 10-15 minutes or until the salmon is cooked through and flakes easily.

For baking, preheat the oven to 375°F (190°C), place the salmon in the baking dish, and cover with foil. Bake for about 15-20 minutes.

2. Prepare the Peas: While the salmon is cooking, if using fresh peas, add them to a small pot of boiling water and cook for about 3-5 minutes until tender. If using frozen peas, you can either boil them for a few minutes or microwave them until warm and soft.

3. Blend the Ingredients: Place the cooked salmon and peas in a blender. Add olive oil and a bit of the cooking water or fish broth to help the blending process.

4. Puree Until Smooth: Blend on high until the mixture is completely smooth. If the puree is too thick, add more water or broth a little at a time until you achieve the desired creamy consistency.

5. Taste the puree and add a pinch of salt if desired. Serve warm, ensuring the texture is suitable for easy swallowing.

Turkey and Sweet Potato Puree

Prep Time: 10 mins | Cook Time: 30 mins | Serves: 2

Per Serving: Calories: 175 | Fat: 4g | Carbs: 15g | Fiber: 3g | Protein: 20g

Ingredients:

- 1/2 pound turkey breast

- 1 cup pumpkin puree (canned or homemade)

- 1/2 cup low-sodium chicken or turkey broth

Procedure:

1. Cook the Turkey: Place the turkey breast in a pot and cover with water. Bring to a boil, then reduce the heat and simmer until the turkey is thoroughly cooked and tender, about 20-25 minutes.

2. Prepare the Pumpkin: If making homemade pumpkin puree, peel and cube fresh pumpkin, steam until soft, and then mash or blend until smooth. If using canned, ensure it's unsweetened and plain.

3. Blend Together: In a blender, combine the cooked turkey, pumpkin puree, and a bit of broth. Blend until smooth, adding more broth as necessary to reach a creamy, smooth consistency.

4. Check the seasoning, adding a little salt if needed. The puree should be completely smooth to make swallowing easy. Serve warm.

Beef and Broccoli Puree

Prep Time: 10 mins | Cook Time: 30 mins | Serves: 2

Per Serving: Calories: 200 | Fat: 8g | Carbs: 10g | Fiber: 3g | Protein: 22g

Ingredients:

- 1/2 pound lean ground beef
- 1 cup broccoli florets
- 1/2 cup beef broth

Procedure:

1. Cook the Beef: In a skillet over medium heat, cook the ground beef until it's fully browned and no longer pink. Drain any excess fat.

2. Steam the Broccoli: Meanwhile, steam the broccoli florets until they are very tender, about 10-15 minutes.

3. Puree the Ingredients: Transfer the cooked beef and broccoli to a blender. Add the beef broth and blend on high until the mixture is completely smooth.

4. Adjust Consistency: If the puree is too thick, add more broth until you reach the desired creamy consistency.

5. Season and Serve: Season with a little salt if necessary, and serve warm, ensuring the texture is smooth and easy to swallow.

Pork and Apple Puree

Prep Time: 10 mins | Cook Time: 25 mins | Serves: 2

Per Serving: Calories: 190 | Fat: 6g | Carbs: 15g | Fiber: 2g | Protein: 18g

Ingredients:

- 1/2 pound pork tenderloin, trimmed

- 2 apples, peeled and cored

- 1/2 cup apple cider or water

Procedure:

1. Cook the Pork: Cut the pork tenderloin into small pieces. In a skillet over medium heat, cook the pork pieces until they are fully cooked and tender, about 15-20 minutes.

2. Prepare the Apples: Chop the peeled and cored apples. In a separate pan, cook the apples with a little water or apple cider until they are soft and mushy, about 10 minutes.

3. Blend Together: Combine the cooked pork and apples in a blender. Add a bit of the cooking liquid from the apples and blend until smooth.

4. Adjust Texture: If the mixture is too thick, add more apple cider or water until the puree reaches a creamy consistency.

5. Taste and add a pinch of cinnamon if desired for extra flavor. Ensure the puree is perfectly smooth for easy swallowing. Serve warm.

Lamb and Mint Puree

Prep Time: 10 mins | Cook Time: 30 mins | Serves: 2

Per Serving: Calories: 220 | Fat: 14g | Carbs: 5g | Fiber: 1g | Protein: 20g

Ingredients:

- 1/2 pound ground lamb
- 1/4 cup mint leaves, finely chopped
- 1/2 cup chicken broth

Procedure:

1. Cook the Lamb: In a skillet, cook the ground lamb over medium heat until it's thoroughly browned and crumbled, about 10 minutes. Drain off any excess fat.

2. Prepare the Mint: While the lamb cooks, finely chop the mint leaves.

3. Blend the Ingredients: Transfer the cooked lamb and chopped mint to a blender. Pour in the chicken broth and blend until smooth.

4. Adjust Consistency: Add more broth if necessary to achieve a smooth, creamy consistency.

5. Check the flavor and add salt if needed. Ensure the texture is suitable for easy swallowing. Serve the puree warm, garnished with additional mint if desired.

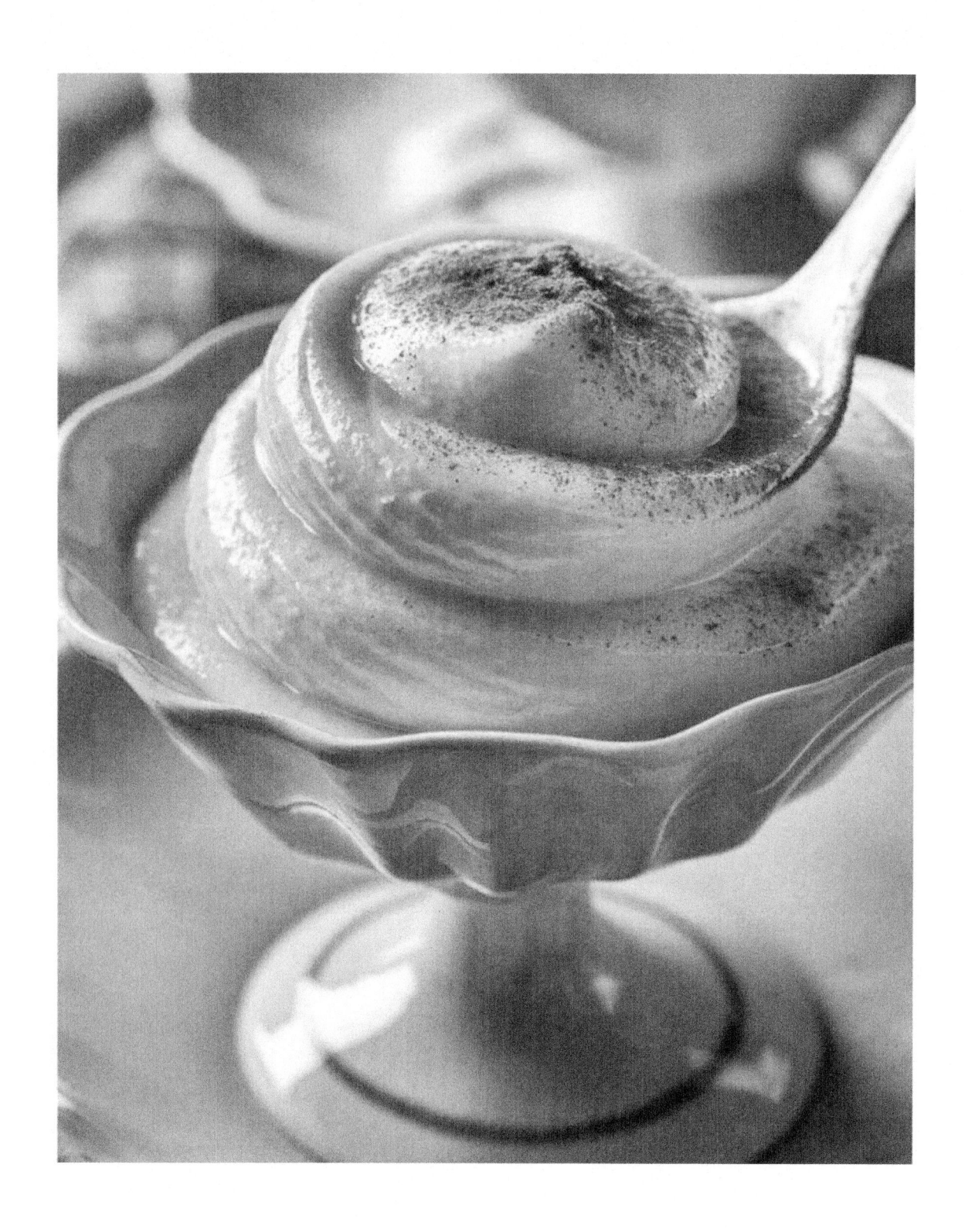

Casseroles and One-Pot Meals

Chicken and Rice Casserole

Prep Time: 10 mins | Cook Time: 45 mins | Serves: 4

Per Serving: Calories: 220 | Fat: 6g | Carbs: 25g | Fiber: 2g | Protein: 18g

Ingredients:

- 2 cups cooked, shredded chicken breast
- 1 cup cooked white rice
- 1 cup cream of chicken soup (ensure it is smooth with no chunks)
- 1/2 cup whole milk
- 1 cup steamed broccoli, finely chopped
- Salt and pepper to taste

Procedure:

1. Preheat the Oven: Preheat your oven to 350°F (175°C).

2. Mix Ingredients: In a large mixing bowl, combine the shredded chicken, cooked rice, cream of chicken soup, milk, and finely chopped broccoli. Stir until well mixed.

3. Season: Add salt and pepper to taste.

4. Bake: Pour the mixture into a greased baking dish. Cover with foil and bake in the preheated oven for 30 minutes.

5. Blend for Smoothness: Once cooked, let the casserole cool slightly, then blend to a smooth, creamy consistency suitable for easy swallowing.

6. Serve warm, ensuring the texture is smooth and uniform.

Salmon and Vegetable Pot Pie

Prep Time: 15 mins | Cook Time: 30 mins | Serves: 4
Per Serving: Calories: 230 | Fat: 10g | Carbs: 20g | Fiber: 3g | Protein: 15g

Ingredients:

- 1 cup cooked salmon, flaked
- 1/2 cup pureed carrots
- 1/2 cup pureed peas
- 1/2 cup cream of celery soup
- 1/4 cup milk
- 1 pre-made pie crust (optional, check consistency)

Procedure:

1. Preheat the Oven: Heat your oven to 375°F (190°C).

2. Combine Ingredients: In a bowl, mix the flaked salmon, pureed carrots, pureed peas, cream of celery soup, and milk.

3. Prepare Pie Crust: If using, lay the pie crust in a pie dish. Ensure the crust is moist enough or omit if not suitable.

4. Fill and Bake: Pour the salmon mixture into the pie crust. Cover with another layer of crust if desired and seal the edges. Bake for about 25-30 minutes until the crust is cooked and the filling is bubbly.

5. Blend for Smoothness: Allow to cool slightly, then blend the filling to ensure it is smooth and easy to swallow.

6. Serve warm, making sure the texture is suitable for dysphagia patients.

Beef and Mashed Potato Casserole

Prep Time: 15 mins | Cook Time: 30 mins | Serves: 4
Per Serving: Calories: 240 | Fat: 8g | Carbs: 25g | Fiber: 3g | Protein: 18g

Ingredients:

- 1/2 pound lean ground beef
- 2 cups mashed potatoes (ensure they are smooth and well-pureed)
- 1 cup pureed mixed vegetables (carrots, peas)
- 1/2 cup low-sodium beef broth
- Salt and pepper to taste

Procedure:

1. Preheat the Oven: Heat your oven to 350°F (175°C).

2. Cook the Beef: In a skillet over medium heat, cook the ground beef until it's thoroughly browned. Drain any excess fat.

3. Prepare the Casserole: In a large mixing bowl, combine the cooked beef, mashed potatoes, and pureed vegetables. Gradually add beef broth to achieve a moist, easily stirrable consistency.

4. Season: Add salt and pepper to taste.

5. Bake: Transfer the mixture to a greased baking dish. Bake in the preheated oven for about 25-30 minutes until the top is slightly golden.

6. Blend for Smoothness: After baking, let the casserole cool slightly, then blend if necessary to achieve a completely smooth consistency.

7. Serve warm, ensuring the texture is appropriate for dysphagia patients.

Turkey and Squash Stew

Prep Time: 10 mins | Cook Time: 40 mins | Serves: 4
Per Serving: Calories: 210 | Fat: 6g | Carbs: 20g | Fiber: 4g | Protein: 20g

Ingredients:

- 1/2 pound turkey breast, cut into small pieces
- 2 cups butternut squash, peeled and cubed
- 1 cup pureed tomatoes
- 1 onion, finely chopped
- 2 cups low-sodium chicken broth
- 1 teaspoon thyme
- Salt and pepper to taste

Procedure:

1. Prepare the Ingredients: Ensure the butternut squash is soft enough to blend easily after cooking.

2. Cook the Stew: In a large pot, sauté the onion until translucent. Add the turkey pieces and cook until no longer pink.

3. Add the Squash and Broth: Add the cubed butternut squash, pureed tomatoes, chicken broth, and thyme. Bring to a boil, then reduce heat and simmer for about 30 minutes, or until the squash is very tender.

4. Blend for Smoothness: Once cooked, use an immersion blender to puree the stew directly in the pot until smooth.

5. Adjust seasoning with salt and pepper. Serve the stew warm, ensuring it has a smooth, creamy texture.

Creamy Chicken and Spinach Bake

Prep Time: 10 mins | Cook Time: 25 mins | Serves: 4
Per Serving: Calories: 220 | Fat: 9g | Carbs: 10g | Fiber: 2g | Protein: 25g

Ingredients:

- 2 cups cooked, shredded chicken breast
- 2 cups spinach, finely chopped and steamed
- 1 cup ricotta cheese
- 1/2 cup low-sodium chicken broth
- Salt and pepper to taste

Procedure:

1. Preheat the Oven: Heat your oven to 350°F (175°C).

2. Mix Ingredients: In a large bowl, combine the shredded chicken, steamed spinach, and ricotta cheese. Mix thoroughly until well combined.

3. Moisten the Mixture: Gradually add chicken broth to the chicken and spinach mixture to achieve a moist, easily stirrable consistency.

4. Season: Add salt and pepper to taste.

5. Bake: Transfer the mixture to a greased baking dish. Cover with foil and bake for 20-25 minutes, until heated through and bubbling.

6. Blend for Smoothness: Allow to cool slightly, then blend if necessary to achieve a completely smooth consistency.

7. Serve warm, ensuring the texture is appropriate for dysphagia patients.

Lentil and Vegetable Pot

Prep Time: 10 mins | Cook Time: 40 mins | Serves: 4
Per Serving: Calories: 180 | Fat: 2g | Carbs: 30g | Fiber: 10g | Protein: 12g

Ingredients:

- 1 cup red lentils
- 2 carrots, peeled and finely chopped
- 2 potatoes, peeled and finely chopped
- 1 onion, finely chopped
- 4 cups vegetable broth
- 1 teaspoon turmeric

- Salt and pepper to taste

Procedure:

1. Prepare Ingredients: Ensure all vegetables are chopped finely enough to blend easily after cooking.

2. Cook the Stew: In a large pot, add the onions and sauté until translucent. Add the chopped carrots, potatoes, red lentils, and vegetable broth.

3. Add Spices: Stir in turmeric and bring the mixture to a boil. Reduce heat and simmer for about 30-35 minutes, or until vegetables and lentils are very soft.

4. Blend for Smoothness: Use an immersion blender to puree the stew directly in the pot until smooth.

5. Adjust seasoning with salt and pepper. Serve the stew warm, ensuring it has a smooth, creamy texture.

Sides and Snacks

Gelatin and Custards

Basic Vanilla Custard

Prep Time: 5 mins | Cook Time: 10 mins | Serves: 4

Per Serving: Calories: 150 | Fat: 5g | Carbs: 20g | Fiber: 0g | Protein: 5g

Ingredients:

- 2 cups milk
- 1/3 cup sugar
- 3 egg yolks
- 1 teaspoon vanilla extract
- 1 tablespoon cornstarch

Procedure:

1. Heat the Milk: In a saucepan, heat the milk and sugar over medium heat until hot but not boiling.

2. Mix Egg Yolks and Cornstarch: In a separate bowl, whisk together the egg yolks and cornstarch until smooth.

3. Temper the Egg Mixture: Slowly pour the hot milk into the egg mixture, whisking constantly to prevent the eggs from scrambling.

4. Cook: Return the mixture to the saucepan and cook over low heat, stirring constantly, until the custard thickens and coats the back of a spoon.

5. Remove from heat, stir in vanilla extract, and pour into serving dishes. Let cool slightly and serve warm, or chill in the refrigerator.

Chocolate Gelatin Dessert

Prep Time: 10 mins | Cook Time: 5 mins | Serves: 4
Per Serving: Calories: 180 | Fat: 3g | Carbs: 35g | Fiber: 1g | Protein: 4g

Ingredients:

- 2 cups water
- 1 packet gelatin powder
- 1/4 cup cocoa powder
- 1/2 cup sugar

Procedure:

1. Dissolve Gelatin: In a small pot, heat one cup of water until hot but not boiling. Add the gelatin powder and stir until completely dissolved.

2. Make Chocolate Mixture: In a separate bowl, mix the cocoa powder and sugar with one cup of cold water until smooth.

3. Add the chocolate mixture to the dissolved gelatin mixture and stir well. Pour into molds or a large dish and refrigerate until set, about 4 hours.

4. Serve: Once set, cut into pieces or scoop to serve.

Lemon Custard

Prep Time: 5 mins | Cook Time: 10 mins | Serves: 4
Per Serving: Calories: 140 | Fat: 4g | Carbs: 22g | Fiber: 0g | Protein: 3g

Ingredients:

- 2 cups milk
- 1/3 cup sugar
- 3 egg yolks
- Zest of 1 lemon
- 1 tablespoon cornstarch
- 2 tablespoons lemon juice

Procedure:

1. Prepare Lemon Zest: Zest one lemon and set aside.

2. Heat the Milk: In a saucepan, combine milk, sugar, and lemon zest. Heat over medium until hot but not boiling.

3. Whisk Egg Yolks and Cornstarch: In a bowl, whisk egg yolks and cornstarch until smooth.

4. Temper and Cook: Gradually add hot milk to the egg mixture, whisking continuously. Return the mixture to the saucepan and cook over low heat, stirring constantly, until the custard thickens.

5. Remove from heat, stir in lemon juice, and pour into serving dishes. Cool slightly and serve warm, or chill if desired.

Mango Gelatin Dessert

Prep Time: 10 mins | Cook Time: 5 mins | Serves: 4
Per Serving: Calories: 120 | Fat: 0g | Carbs: 30g | Fiber: 1g | Protein: 2g

Ingredients:

- 2 cups mango juice
- 1 packet gelatin powder
- 1/2 cup diced ripe mango

Procedure:

1. Dissolve Gelatin: Heat one cup of mango juice in a small pot until just about to boil. Remove from heat and whisk in the gelatin powder until completely dissolved.

2. Mix: In a bowl, combine the dissolved gelatin mixture with the remaining one cup of cold mango juice. Stir well.

3. Add Mango: Fold in the diced mango, then pour the mixture into molds or a dish.

4. Refrigerate until firm, about 4 hours. Serve chilled, ensuring the texture is smooth and suitable for swallowing.

Strawberry Custard

Prep Time: 10 mins | Cook Time: 10 mins | Serves: 4
Per Serving: Calories: 160 | Fat: 5g | Carbs: 25g | Fiber: 1g | Protein: 4g

Ingredients:

- 2 cups milk
- 1/3 cup sugar
- 3 egg yolks
- 1 cup pureed strawberries
- 1 tablespoon cornstarch

Procedure:

1. Heat the Milk: In a saucepan, combine the milk and sugar and heat over medium until hot but not boiling.

2. Mix Egg Yolks and Cornstarch: In a separate bowl, whisk together the egg yolks and cornstarch.

3. Temper the Egg Mixture: Slowly pour the hot milk into the egg mixture, whisking constantly to prevent the eggs from scrambling.

4. Cook the Custard: Return the mixture to the saucepan and cook over low heat, stirring constantly, until the custard thickens.

5. Stir in the strawberry puree until well combined. Pour the custard into serving dishes, let cool slightly, and serve warm or chill in the refrigerator.

Coffee Gelatin Dessert

Prep Time: 5 mins | Cook Time: 5 mins | Serves: 4
Per Serving: Calories: 100 | Fat: 0g | Carbs: 24g | Fiber: 0g | Protein: 2g

Ingredients:

- 2 cups strong brewed coffee
- 1 packet gelatin powder
- 1/4 cup sugar

Procedure:

1. Prepare Coffee: Brew 2 cups of strong coffee.
2. Dissolve Gelatin and Sugar: Heat the brewed coffee just to boiling and remove from heat. Stir in the gelatin powder and sugar until completely dissolved.
3. Set: Pour the coffee mixture into molds or a shallow dish.
4. Refrigerate until set, about 3-4 hours. Serve chilled, ensuring the texture is smooth and easy to swallow.

Peach Gelatin Dessert

Prep Time: 10 mins | Cook Time: 5 mins | Serves: 4
Per Serving: Calories: 110 | Fat: 0g | Carbs: 28g | Fiber: 1g | Protein: 2g

Ingredients:

- 2 cups peach juice

- 1 packet gelatin powder

- 1/2 cup finely diced fresh peaches

Procedure:

1. Dissolve Gelatin: In a saucepan, heat one cup of peach juice until it is just about to boil. Remove from heat and whisk in the gelatin powder until completely dissolved.

2. Combine: Stir in the remaining one cup of cold peach juice along with the diced peaches.

3. Pour the mixture into molds or a serving dish and refrigerate until firm, about 4 hours. Ensure the gelatin is completely set and smooth before serving.

Blueberry Custard

Prep Time: 10 mins | Cook Time: 10 mins | Serves: 4

Per Serving: Calories: 170 | Fat: 5g | Carbs: 27g | Fiber: 2g | Protein: 4g

Ingredients:

- 2 cups milk

- 1/3 cup sugar

- 3 egg yolks

- 1 cup blueberry puree (ensure it is smooth)

- 1 tablespoon cornstarch

Procedure:

1. Prepare the Milk: In a saucepan, heat the milk and sugar over medium heat until it is hot but not boiling.

2. Mix Egg Yolks and Cornstarch: In a separate bowl, thoroughly whisk together the egg yolks and cornstarch.

3. Temper the Egg Mixture: Gradually add the hot milk to the egg mixture, whisking constantly to prevent the eggs from scrambling.

4. Cook the Custard: Return the mixture to the saucepan and cook over low heat, stirring constantly, until the custard thickens and can coat the back of a spoon.

5. Add Blueberry Puree and Serve: Stir in the blueberry puree until well combined. Pour into serving dishes, let cool slightly, and serve warm or chill if preferred.

Raspberry Gelatin Dessert

Prep Time: 10 mins | Cook Time: 5 mins | Serves: 4

Per Serving: Calories: 100 | Fat: 0g | Carbs: 25g | Fiber: 2g | Protein: 2g

Ingredients:

- 2 cups water

- 1 packet gelatin powder

- 1/2 cup sugar

- 1 cup raspberry puree (strained to remove seeds)

Procedure:

1. Prepare Gelatin Base: In a saucepan, heat the water to a near boil. Remove from heat and whisk in the gelatin and sugar until both are completely dissolved.

2. Add Raspberry Puree: Stir in the raspberry puree until the mixture is smooth.

3. Pour the mixture into molds or a shallow dish. Refrigerate until set, about 3-4 hours. Serve chilled, ensuring it is smooth and easy to swallow.

Caramel Custard

Prep Time: 15 mins | Cook Time: 35 mins | Serves: 4

Per Serving: Calories: 220 | Fat: 7g | Carbs: 35g | Fiber: 0g | Protein: 5

Ingredients:

- 2 cups milk

- 1/2 cup sugar, plus 1/4 cup for caramel

- 3 egg yolks

- 1 teaspoon vanilla extract

Procedure:

1. Prepare Caramel: In a saucepan, heat 1/4 cup of sugar over medium heat until it melts and becomes amber in color. Carefully pour the hot caramel into the bottom of each serving dish.

2. Heat the Milk: In another saucepan, warm the milk but do not boil.

3. Whisk Eggs and Sugar: In a bowl, whisk the egg yolks with 1/2 cup sugar until smooth.

4. Combine and Cook: Gradually add the hot milk to the egg mixture, stirring continuously. Return the mixture to the heat and cook gently until it thickens.

5. Bake: Pour the custard mixture over the caramel in the dishes. Place the dishes in a water bath and bake in a preheated oven at 350°F (175°C) for about 25 minutes.

6. Cool and Serve: Let the custard cool, then refrigerate until set. Serve chilled.

Chapter 6: Beverages and Smoothies

Thickened Drinks for Hydration

High-Protein Vanilla Shake

- *Ingredients:*

  - 1 cup whole milk

  - 1 scoop vanilla protein powder

  - 1/2 banana

  - 1 tablespoon honey (optional for sweetness)

  - 1-2 teaspoons commercial thickener (adjust based on desired consistency)

Procedure:

1. Prepare Ingredients: Measure all your ingredients before starting. Peel the half banana and break it into smaller chunks to make blending easier.

2. Blend Smoothly: Place the milk, vanilla protein powder, and banana chunks into a blender. If you like your shake a bit sweeter, add the tablespoon of honey.

3. Blend Until Smooth: Blend the ingredients on high speed for about 30-45 seconds or until the mixture is completely smooth.

4. Add Thickener: With the blender off, add 1 teaspoon of commercial thickener. Blend again for 15-20 seconds, check the consistency, and if needed, add another teaspoon of thickener.

5. Check Consistency: The shake should be smooth and thick enough to ensure safe swallowing. Adjust thickness by adding more thickener if necessary.

6. Serve Immediately: Pour the shake into a glass and serve immediately to maintain its freshness and texture.

Nutrient-Dense Berry Smoothie

Ingredients:

- 1 cup almond milk or soy milk
- 1/2 cup mixed berries (strawberries, blueberries, raspberries), fresh or frozen
- 1 scoop protein powder
- 1-2 teaspoons commercial thickener

Procedure:

1. Prepare Ingredients: If using frozen berries, measure out 1/2 cup and let them sit at room temperature for a few minutes to slightly thaw for easier blending.

2. Combine Ingredients in Blender: Add the almond or soy milk, berries, and protein powder to the blender.

3. Blend Until Smooth: Blend on high for about 1 minute or until the mixture is very smooth, ensuring there are no chunks left.

4. Thicken the Smoothie: Add 1 teaspoon of thickener and blend for another 20 seconds. Check the thickness and add more thickener if needed.

5. Serve: Once the desired consistency is reached, pour the smoothie into a glass and serve immediately.

Creamy Avocado and Spinach Shake

Ingredients:

 - 1/2 ripe avocado

 - 1 cup spinach leaves, fresh

 - 1 cup coconut milk

 - 1 scoop protein powder

 - 1-2 teaspoons commercial thickener

Procedure:

1. Prepare the Avocado: Cut the avocado in half, remove the pit, and scoop out the flesh with a spoon.

2. Ready Ingredients: Rinse the spinach leaves under cold water to clean any residue or grit.

3. Blend Ingredients: Place the avocado, spinach, coconut milk, and protein powder into a blender.

4. Blend Until Very Smooth: Blend the mixture on high for about 1 to 2 minutes, ensuring all components are fully pureed and the texture is completely smooth.

5. Add Thickener: Incorporate the thickener and blend again for 20-30 seconds. Check the consistency and adjust by adding more thickener if needed.

6. Serve: Pour the shake into a glass and serve right away to enjoy its full flavor and creamy texture.

Peanut Butter Banana Shake

Ingredients:

- 1 cup whole milk
- 1 ripe banana
- 2 tablespoons peanut butter
- 1 scoop protein powder (optional)
- 1-2 teaspoons commercial thickener

Procedure:

1. Prepare the Banana: Peel the banana and cut it into small pieces to make it easier to blend.

2. Blend the Ingredients: In a blender, combine the whole milk, banana pieces, peanut butter, and protein powder if using. Blend on high until the mixture is completely smooth.

3. Thicken the Shake: With the blender turned off, add 1 teaspoon of the commercial thickener. Blend again for about 20 seconds, then check the consistency. If needed, add more thickener and blend again.

4. Final Consistency Check: Ensure the shake is smooth and thick enough for easy swallowing. Adjust the thickness by adding more thickener if necessary.

5. Serve: Pour the shake into a glass and serve immediately to ensure freshness and the right texture for easy swallowing.

Creamy Mango Smoothie

Ingredients:

- 1 cup mango chunks, fresh or frozen

- 1 cup coconut milk

- 1 tablespoon honey (optional, for extra sweetness)

- 1-2 teaspoons commercial thickener

Procedure:

1. Prepare Mango: If using frozen mango, let the chunks sit out for a few minutes to thaw slightly for easier blending.

2. Combine Ingredients: In a blender, add the mango chunks and coconut milk. If desired, add honey for additional sweetness.

3. Blend Until Smooth: Blend on high for about 1 minute or until the smoothie is completely smooth.

4. Add Thickener: Incorporate the thickener into the smoothie while the blender is off, then blend for an additional 20-30 seconds. Check the consistency and add more thickener if needed.

5. Serve: Once the smoothie has reached the desired thickness, pour it into a glass and serve immediately.

Avocado Cucumber Shake

Ingredients:

- 1/2 ripe avocado
- 1/2 cucumber, peeled and sliced
- 1 cup plain yogurt or kefir
- 1-2 teaspoons commercial thickener

Procedure:

1. Prepare the Ingredients: Scoop the avocado flesh out of its skin and slice the cucumber into thin pieces.

2. Blend the Ingredients: In a blender, combine the avocado, cucumber, and yogurt or kefir. Blend on high until the mixture is completely smooth.

3. Thicken the Shake: Add the thickener to the blender and mix until it is fully incorporated and the shake reaches a suitable consistency for swallowing.

4. Consistency Check and Serve: Check that the shake is smooth and not too thick or thin. Adjust by adding more thickener or a little water if necessary. Serve immediately, ensuring it is at a comfortable temperature for consumption.

Flavorful Smoothie and Juice

Classic Green Juice

ingredients:

- 1 cup spinach

- 1 green apple, cored

- 1/2 cucumber

- 1 stalk celery

- Juice of 1/2 lemon

Procedure:

1. Thoroughly rinse spinach, apple, cucumber, and celery.

2. Core the apple and slice along with cucumber and celery to fit your juicer.

3. Juice the ingredients, starting with spinach, followed by apple, cucumber, and celery.

4. Squeeze the lemon juice into the mix and stir well.

5. Serve the juice immediately to maximize nutrient intake.

Beetroot and Carrot Juice

Ingredients:

- 1 beetroot, peeled

- 2 carrots, peeled

- 1/2 inch ginger

- Juice of 1/2 orange

Procedure:

1. Peel and chop beetroot and carrots into juicer-friendly pieces.

2. Juice beetroot, carrots, and ginger together.

3. Stir in the freshly squeezed orange juice for additional sweetness and vitamin C.

4. Serve the juice fresh for optimal flavor and nutritional benefits.

Tropical Mango Juice

Ingredients:

- 1 ripe mango, peeled and pit removed

- 1/2 cup pineapple chunks

- Juice of 1 lime

Procedure:

1. Prepare the mango and pineapple by cutting them into pieces suitable for juicing or blending.

2. Juice or blend the fruits until smooth.

3. Add the lime juice and mix well.

4. Serve chilled for a refreshing and hydrating drink.

Refreshing Watermelon Juice

Ingredients:

- 2 cups watermelon, cubed and seeds removed

- Juice of 1/2 lime

- Mint leaves for garnish

- *Procedure*:

1. Blend the watermelon cubes until smooth.

2. Optionally strain through a fine mesh for a smoother texture.

3. Stir in the lime juice and mix thoroughly.

4. Garnish with fresh mint leaves and serve chilled.

Immune Boosting Orange Juice

Ingredients:

- 3 oranges, peeled

- 1/2 inch turmeric root or 1/2 teaspoon turmeric powder

- 1/2 inch ginger root

Procedure:

1. Juice the peeled oranges, turmeric, and ginger together.

2. Ensure all ingredients are thoroughly juiced and mixed.

3. Serve the juice immediately to enjoy its full immune-boosting benefits.

Antioxidant Berry Juice

Ingredients:

- 1 cup mixed berries (strawberries, blueberries, raspberries)

- 1 apple, cored

Procedure:

1. If using a juicer, first process the apple, followed by the berries to extract maximum juice.

2. If using a blender, combine both fruits and blend until smooth, then strain if desired to remove the seeds.

3. Serve the juice immediately to take advantage of the antioxidants in the berries.

Carrot Apple Ginger Juice

Ingredients:

- 3 carrots, peeled

- 2 apples, cored

- 1-inch piece of ginger, peeled

Procedure:

1. Chop the carrots and apples into sizes suitable for your juicer.

2. Start by juicing the ginger, followed by carrots and apples.

3. Stir the juice well to mix the flavors.

4. Serve immediately to enjoy its invigorating taste and nutritional benefits.

Chapter 7

Meal plan

Day 1: - Breakfast: Silky Rice Pudding Berry Parfait with Whipped Cream - Lunch: Pureed Butternut Squash Soup - Dinner: Scrambled Eggs or Omelet with Soft Buns or Pancakes	Day 2: - Breakfast: Soft Pancakes (Classic) - Lunch: Creamy Mashed Potatoes - Dinner: Meatloaf or Casserole (No Chunks) with Well-Cooked Vegetables
Day 3: - Breakfast: Chilled Mango Mousse - Lunch: Silky Carrot and Ginger Soup - Dinner: Soft Chicken and Rice	Day 4: - Breakfast: Cream of Wheat with Cinnamon - Lunch: Mashed Sweet Potatoes - Dinner: Gentle Fish Chowder
Day 5: - Breakfast: Soft Scrambled Tofu - Lunch: Pureed Lentil Soup	Day 6: - Breakfast: Banana Pancakes (Oatmeal Banana Pancakes)

- Dinner: Tender Beef Stew with Soft Vegetables	- Lunch: Soft Rice Casserole with Vegetables - Dinner: Soft Spinach and Cheese Quiche
Day 7: - Breakfast: Yogurt Pancakes - Lunch: Creamy Pumpkin Risotto - Dinner: Soft Chicken and Mushroom Risotto	**Day 8:** - Breakfast: Ricotta Cheese Pancakes - Lunch: Soft Quinoa Salad with Avocado - Dinner: Smooth Pumpkin Risotto
Day 9: - Breakfast: Pumpkin Spice Pancakes - Lunch: Pureed Broccoli and Cheddar Soup - Dinner: Soft Cauliflower Mash	**Day 10:** - Breakfast: Apple Cinnamon Pancakes - Lunch: Soft Tofu Stir-Fry - Dinner: Scrambled Eggs or Omelet with Soft Buns or Pancakes
Day 11: - Breakfast: Blueberry Yogurt Pancakes - Lunch: Creamy Cauliflower Soup - Dinner: Meatloaf or Casserole (No Chunks) with Well-Cooked Vegetables	**Day 12:** - Breakfast: Silken Scrambled Eggs - Lunch: Mashed Potatoes or Squash - Dinner: Gentle Fish Chowder

Day 13:	**Day 14:**
- Breakfast: Egg Custard	- Breakfast: Basic Vanilla Custard
- Lunch: Pureed Lentil Curry	- Lunch: Soft Spinach and Cheese Quiche
- Dinner: Tender Beef Stew with Soft Vegetables	- Dinner: Soft Chicken and Rice

Conclusion

Coping wwith dysphagia can be challenging, not just for the individual diagnosed but also for their families and caregivers. The " Dysphagia Cookbook" has been meticulously crafted to ease this transition, offering not just recipes but a new perspective on food and its preparation. Our goal has been to restore the joy of eating without compromising safety or nutrition.

This cookbook serves as more than just a collection of recipes—it's a guide to understanding how texture, consistency, and nutritional balance play crucial roles in managing dysphagia. Each recipe has been tailored to meet specific needs, ensuring that meals are easy to swallow, highly nutritious, and appealing. From breakfast smoothies and hearty soups to nutrient-packed dinners and delightful desserts, we have strived to bring variety and flavor back to the table.

Moreover, the educational content within this book aims to empower readers with knowledge about dysphagia. It provides insights into how different consistencies can aid in easier swallowing and how to adjust meals to individual requirements effectively. We also discussed the importance of staying hydrated with suitable drinks and how to use commercial thickeners properly.

In crafting these meals, we have focused on using accessible ingredients that can be easily transformed into soft, appetizing meals that cater to both taste and health needs. We hope this cookbook becomes a trusted companion in your kitchen, helping to make mealtime a pleasurable and safe experience once again.

As you use this cookbook, remember that the journey with dysphagia is highly individual. What works for one person may not work for another, so feel encouraged to experiment with the consistency and flavors based on specific preferences and medical advice.

Finally, this cookbook is not just about adapting to a new way of eating—it's about embracing change with positivity and creativity. With each page, we hope to inspire confidence in the kitchen, offering ways to innovate and adapt recipes that will nourish both body and spirit.

"Thank you for reading! I hope you found inspiration in these pages to take control of your dysphagia diagnosis and rediscover the pleasure of eating. Wishing you a lifetime of delicious and safe meals!"

MY WEEKLY MEAL PLANNER

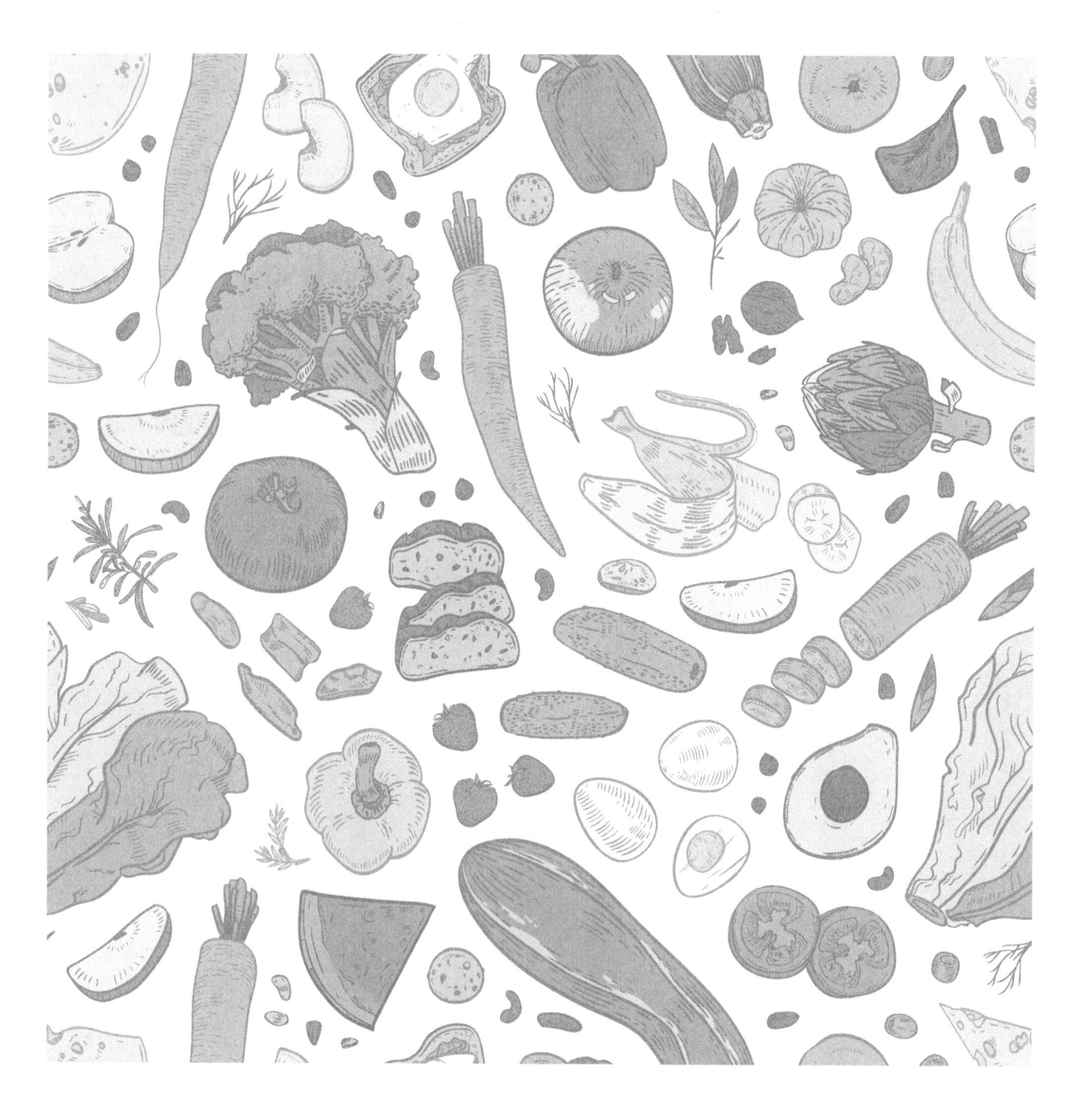

Meal planner

Dates _____

	BREAKFAST	LUNCH	DINNER	SNACKS
MON				
TUE				
WED				
THU				
FRI				
SAT				
SUN				

Shopping list

_____
_____
_____
_____
_____

_____
_____
_____
_____
_____

Note:

_____
_____
_____
_____
_____

Meal planner

Dates _____

	BREAKFAST	LUNCH	DINNER	SNACKS
MON				
TUE				
WED				
THU				
FRI				
SAT				
SUN				

Shopping list

_____
_____
_____
_____

_____
_____
_____
_____

Note:

_____
_____
_____
_____

Meal planner

Dates _____

	BREAKFAST	LUNCH	DINNER	SNACKS
MON				
TUE				
WED				
THU				
FRI				
SAT				
SUN				

Shopping list

_____ _____

_____ _____

_____ _____

_____ _____

_____ _____

Note:

_____

_____

_____

_____

_____

Meal planner

Dates _____

	BREAKFAST	LUNCH	DINNER	SNACKS
MON				
TUE				
WED				
THU				
FRI				
SAT				
SUN				

Shopping list

_____

_____

_____

_____

_____

Note:

_____

_____

_____

_____

_____

Meal planner

Dates _____

	BREAKFAST	LUNCH	DINNER	SNACKS
MON				
TUE				
WED				
THU				
FRI				
SAT				
SUN				

Shopping list

_____
_____
_____
_____
_____

_____
_____
_____
_____
_____

Note:

_____
_____
_____
_____
_____

Meal planner

Dates _____

	BREAKFAST	LUNCH	DINNER	SNACKS
MON				
TUE				
WED				
THU				
FRI				
SAT				
SUN				

Shopping list

_____
_____
_____
_____
_____

_____
_____
_____
_____
_____

Note:

_____
_____
_____
_____
_____

Meal planner

Dates _____

	BREAKFAST	LUNCH	DINNER	SNACKS
MON				
TUE				
WED				
THU				
FRI				
SAT				
SUN				

Shopping list

_____ _____

_____ _____

_____ _____

_____ _____

Note:

_____

_____

_____

_____

Meal planner

Dates _____

	BREAKFAST	LUNCH	DINNER	SNACKS
MON				
TUE				
WED				
THU				
FRI				
SAT				
SUN				

Shopping list

_____
_____
_____
_____
_____

_____
_____
_____
_____
_____

Note:

_____
_____
_____
_____
_____

Printed in Dunstable, United Kingdom